# WHAT
# *70 Plus Years*
# HAVE TAUGHT ME
# ABOUT HEALTH
# AND FITNESS

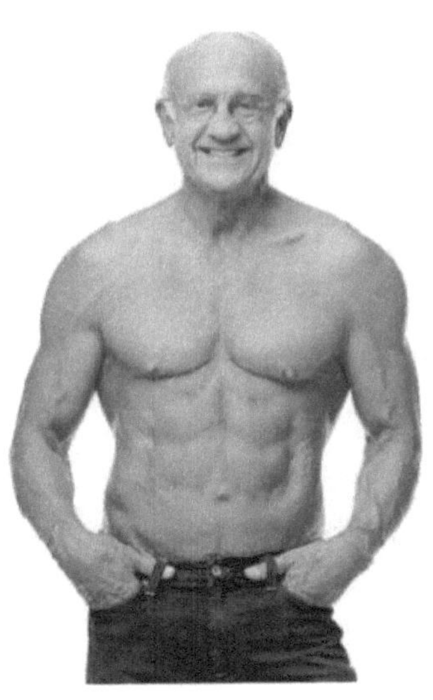

*Figure 1 The Amazing Dr Jeffry Life Aged 73*

# TABLE OF CONTENTS

# About The Author

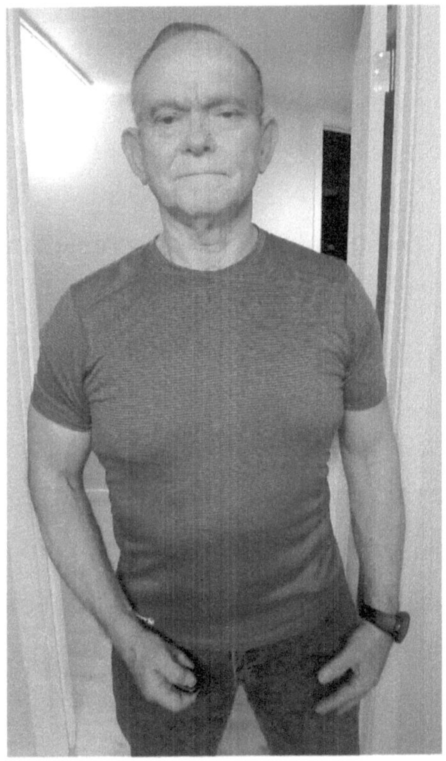

*Figure 2 The Author aged 71 in 2018*

I have learned about aging in my past 71 years. I actually started earlier than most men when in the 1980's (my late 30's and early 40's) I took a serious approach to supplements especially anti-oxidants and Sun Tan lotion, Sun Tan lotion all the time.

Then in the 90's (my early 50's I started taking a closer look at skin care. In my 60's I began to get serious about my diet and nutrition and exercise.

This book is dedicated to sharing with others what I have learned over those decades. My primary interest is in providing helpful information to those men over 60 but it is never too soon to begin caring about how you age.

In fact the earlier you start the longer the techniques I have learned will have to make a difference. For those over 60 it is never too late to get started. Don't wait any longer, because the longer you wait the harder it will be to correct previous damage your body has accumulated over your life.

What makes me an expert on the subject of anti-aging you ask? The answer is nothing. My intent is not to prove myself any kind of expert but to share with others what my life's journey and research has shown me. I believe some of the things I have tried really have worked for me.

There are a lot of factors that go into aging such as fitness, diet and nutrition, lifestyle and others. But if you asked me which was the most important I would have to say diet and nutrition.

The others are important but diet and nutrition are the most important. Hence this will be the main focus of this site. Excuse this much over used cliche but "We are what we eat."

Remember that I'm only a normal individual like you. I'm energetic about this stuff, however I don't have a PhD in gerontology or even a degree in medicine. The data in this book is readily out there for anybody with the get up and go to look for it. I urge you to do your own studies too and make your own conclusions.

Thurman Ray Plumlee

www.Over60Health.info

# INTRODUCTION

There is now no doubt about it. Health and Fitness for older adults has many benefits. It was not too long ago (At least it does not seem that long ago.) back in the 1950's when doctors felt strenuous exercise for older men would stress the heart and cause life threatening damage. Well, we have come a long way.

For the purpose of this BOOK, I am going to focus on health and fitness benefits for us old folks. Whether you use soup cans, weights, machines, resistance bands, isometrics (my favorite) or body weight exercises. Health and fitness training for senior men is critical if we want to live a vibrant and active retirement.

It really does not matter how old you are or whether you are confined to a wheel chair or bed. Exercise is one of the factors that help in improving the health and quality of life, especially for a senior citizen.

No matter what age you are and even if you have never exercised in your young days, you can always start at any point of time. It has been proved that there are many benefits of exercising in old age, as most seniors have started taking it seriously and living longer and healthier.

The aspects that need to be considered when wanting to exercise more are seeking medical advice for health checkups, anti-aging care, nutritional supplementation, diet, and utilizing time.

With age the muscle mass in the body decreases. Muscle is important for the body in many ways because it keeps the body strong and burns the calories so that the body weight can be maintained. It also contributes to bone strength and balance of the body.

The muscles of the body are interrelated to the neurological system of the body. If you want to perform any action with your muscles, the brain first processes the thought. It then sends signals to the muscles which need to move and perform the action.

As one grows older the body's system slows down, movements and reflexes slow down too, immunity reduces and healing is also slow. However, science has discovered ways to help the body to renew itself and make it easy to get the energy to participate in an invigorating exercise routine.

It is interesting to note that if you start exercising, for example by joining a weight-lifting program, the muscle patterning improves, even though there is no increase in the muscle mass. Hence exercises can be beneficial for seniors as they can get stronger without building big muscles.

Walking is the commonest exercise recommended for seniors, as walking burns the fat in your body. A simple-to-use step counter could be a part of your daily fitness program, just to add to your weight loss plan and get rid of unwanted fat. Walking generally helps you to get better sleep, so that you can wake up fresh the next morning.

A senior should make walking a part of everyday life; it will contribute to your overall health. Join in trails or walking programs organized by your community. It can be exercise as well as fun for all the seniors. Another idea is to start a walking group, where people of the same age group can walk together.

Strength exercises for seniors should be done with care, especially if one is starting for the first time. Go slow and build up step by step, so that you don't lose confidence and give it up totally. There are certain safety tips which every senior should be aware of.

While doing strength exercises in a fitness center, concentrate on your breathing. You should never hold your breath, as it may affect the blood pressure. The body is not agile, so don't use jerking and thrusting movements, just make the movements smooth and steady. The muscles may remain sore for a few days and there may be slight fatigue as well.

But there should not be exhaustion and sore joints. If painful muscle pulls should occur, the exercises are not being done properly. Muscle exercises are otherwise helpful for men, whereas brisk walks help aging women to reduce anxiety, stress and depression.

To maintain optimal health, it is wise to benefit from the many different ways your diet can be supplemented. You may need to support optimal organ and tissue function with products that have been scientifically proven in clinical studies.

Before starting any exercise program consult a doctor and/or a dietician, so that your state of health can be checked and you can regulate your meals and diet according to their advice. Eat the food that suits your body, and not the food that makes you sick, even though you may enjoy it.

Happy Reading.

# CHAPTER 1

## *FOREVER EATING: WHY EATING CONSUMES US AND DESTROYS US*

The foods that one consumes on a daily basis can greatly affect one's health in so many ways. Although fast food is convenient, it is not the best for one's longevity and overall wellbeing. People are usually pushed into eating a healthy diet because of health scares such as heart attacks or cancer.

The risk of developing diseases is so much higher in people that have unhealthy diets. For this reason, it is very important that people adopt healthier eating habits. Not only will it lower the chances of developing life threatening illnesses; it will also help to improve a person's wellbeing each day.

One of the main reasons people should eat a healthy diet is to prevent and fight disease. When people consume foods that are very unhealthy they place their overall health in jeopardy. People that eat foods that are high in fat are more likely to develop heart disease and to be overweight.

It is very important to realize that the foods that one consumes can either benefit health or destroy it. The choice is up to the individual. Instead of eating loads of sugary snacks that have very little nutritional value, people can satisfy their sweet tooth with fruit which is not only good for preventing and fighting certain diseases, it also can keep a person's weight down.

Instead of eating foods such as chips, pastries and candies which do not have any nutritional value whatsoever, it is better to eat fruits, vegetables and lean meats and fish. All of these healthy food options contain vitamins, minerals and other substances that will support healthy bodily function while preventing a number of major diseases.

An additional reason it is important to eat a healthy diet is that it prevents weight gain and obesity. One of the main reasons there are so many people that are struggling with their weight is because of their diets. Many people with weight issues are not adopting a lifestyle where they eat healthy foods in moderation coupled with regular physical activity.

Eating the healthy foods is very important for keeping one's weight down. It can be very difficult to lose or maintain one's weight if the foods consumed are high in fat and calories. Likewise, the ways in which foods are prepared play a major role in obesity.

Such methods of preparing food as frying can make even the best food incredibly unhealthy. Eating a healthy diet is the best way to lower one's weight and prevent the many health concerns that are a result of being overweight.

A healthy diet improves mental functioning. This should not come as a surprise since there are many good foods such as fish that are high in nutrients such as omega-3 fatty acids. Such substances are very important in promoting the function of the brain. Studies have shown that eating foods that are high in saturated fats can have a change the way the brain operates.

This occurs as a result of the cell membranes of the brain become less flexible. Thus, it pays to eat healthy in order to increase mental functioning.

Overall, the importance of eating healthy foods cannot be underestimated. People should consider the positive effects that a juicy peach or crunchy carrot will have on their bodies the next time they get a craving for pastries and chips.

Eating right is always a necessity, that when coupled with a workout program will be highly beneficial. Your diet must include healthy dietary fats that are needed for the cell membranes that are within your body.

Healthy foods allow your body cells to function normally. But bad foods can destroy your body cells. Foods that are processed and chemically treated will break down your cellular structure from lack of proper nutrition. Your cells will either be destroyed or be damaged, forcing other cells to compensate. When this happens, diseases do occur.

Healthy eating creates a balanced body. Hormone production is normal. Muscle building occurs at a normal rate and fat burning occurs. The vitamins and minerals our body consumes are absorbed and used for enzyme regulation.

The reason we don't eat right is because it is hard to do. Most healthy food is expensive and most stores sell foods that are processed and full of junk. We buy those foods because of the taste rather than the nutritional value of them.

The second reason is we were deceived to believe that good fats (those that are natural and unprocessed) have been removed from foods when we actually need those types of fat. And the third reason is because we as a society have become too lazy.

We eat out constantly and restaurants we go to do not use the proper oils to cook with. They always go for the cheapest foods that are processed and unhealthy. Developing a healthy body takes much dedication. We need to watch what we eat before we end up destroying ourselves.

# CHAPTER 2

## *SOCIAL CENTERPIECE OF OUR DAILY LIFE*

We can't avoid events such as family gatherings, parties, get togethers, and others that involve our social life. We have to face it, we need these events in order to have a social life and survive this world.

Occasions such as these always have a variety of foods and drinks to choose from, and it's hard to face away from temptation. It's so easy to be tempted to eat anything you want when you're at parties and you can always find an excuse to eat them.

I hate to break this to you, but if you really want to lose weight, this can't help. I can give you tips on how to eat out with friends the healthy way.

You can have fun and be with your friends and family at the same time still maintain your diet. Just think of the models and celebrities who have endless parties to attend to but are still able to stay in shape. Events like these are part of their work and social networking that can help survive their career.

Before going to a party or event, drink a cup of green tea or Perrier with a slice of lemon. It will help reduce your appetite. This way, it's going to be easier when you're at buffets, because you're going to pick the smallest plate available.

Another tip is order an appetizer instead of the main course. Don't worry, you'll still feel full because portions of appetizers have grown. Don't order fried foods and dishes with sauce;

if you're in an Italian restaurant, order dishes that have tomato-based sauce.

When you're at a cocktail party, avoid samosas, chicken nuggets, and anything fried or covered in sauce. Drink a diet Coke with your cocktail to control your appetite. Do your socializing as far away from the snacks table as possible. Aim for the vegetables like the hummus platter, with carrot and celery to dip.

Alcoholic drinks are extremely hard to avoid in parties. So, you can still drink alcohol, but choose light beers because they have fewer calories. Order your drinks with soda instead of tonic, since tonic is high in calories.

Stay away from fruit juices because they are full of sugar. Try diet Coke as mixer for your drink and a white wine spritzer, I hear it tastes great during summer. Drink your wine after your meal rather than beforehand, because wine can stimulate your appetite.

Not only does fasting for long hours before a big holiday dinner slow metabolic rates, but you may end up going to the party overly hungry and end up overeating. Eat small meals and have healthy snacks before a big holiday dinner so that you don't attend the party feeling famished.

Control Dinner Party Choices

Pick up a small plate to help control portion sizes and fill it up with healthy appetizers, salad, and vegetables if they are available. You don't have to sacrifice favorite snacks at holiday parties.

Satisfy a craving with a few small bites, and don't go back for seconds on richer foods. For dinner, limit or avoid cream sauces, cheesy dips, gravy, and butter. Savor the food at parties by eating slow. This gives your brain time to receive the signal that your stomach is full.

Watch the Drinks

Alcoholic beverages contain a lot of calories, and some more than others. Besides limiting your alcohol intake to one or two servings, pay attention to the type of drinks you have.

Specialty cocktails can be replaced with a light beer or wine. In addition, alternating between alcoholic and calorie free non-alcoholic drinks helps to pace yourself and stay hydrated.

Know When To Say NO

People often feel forced to eat because good natured relatives and friends keep placing more food on their plate. Others may want you to take home leftovers. It is okay to politely decline even the most insistent of relatives and friends.

Many people look at a party as a food event, but there is more to a holiday party than food. Parties are also about celebrating and enjoying good times in the company of your friends and family. If you find yourself standing around the food table, start a conversation to divert your attention from the food.

Food

Use a small plate; you can always go for a second helping if you want some more later.

Balance your plate: 1 portion (size of your palm) of protein i.e. Turkey, 1 portion of potatoes/stuffing, and have a plate of veg and sprouts.

Dessert: Just have one, not three. Christmas Cake: Don't have a piece the size of a large boot.

Chips/Crisps: Balance with healthy dips like hummus or guacamole, carrots, cucumber, cauliflower and broccoli. Make the most of the cake, pies and crisps; they can probably be a meal in themselves, so if you plan them at the right time, you might not need much else if you've had a massive meal that day.

Alcohol

Put Food Away: When you drink you lose all sense of discernment about what you're going to eat. So, put those nibbles/crisps etc away after an hour.

Use Mixers: Hang overs are the worst, so add fizzy water to your wine (or lemonade), or drink water in between each drink.

Have 'dry days': Have days off from drinking during the Christmas holiday, plan them now.

Be prepared: Get some sports drinks or Resolve in for the next day.

In life most of the decisions we make are driven by our subconscious mind more so than our conscious mind. Often the things we do are not done from a position of strength but rather from a position of weakness. This is especially true in the area of food.

If you were to observe how you behave around food on a daily basis, you would see this to be true. Ask yourself, how often you eat because you are genuinely hungry versus simply eating because food is present. As you continue to read below you will discover 3 significant reasons why you eat what you do and when you do.

If we are honest with ourselves, many times we eat for the simple joy of food. I am sure we can all agree that certain foods taste really good and we derive great pleasure in consuming them. While on the surface this may not be a bad thing, if you are battling health issues or weight gain, it is important that this desire for eating for eating sake be controlled.

Have you ever been invited to a party or an event and purchased food even though you had just eaten before arriving? We see it all the time at birthday parties. It almost seems offensive to sit at a table where others are eating and you have nothing in front of you.

Not only are you uncomfortable, your table mates are equally uncomfortable. They offer to buy you something just so they don't have to eat alone. To live a vibrant and healthy lifestyle, having the courage to not participate in this is crucial.

We are all guilty of relieving our stress through food. I find it amazing how much happiness a small piece of candy can bring.

At times this is not so bad however when eating becomes the primary way you relieve stress, you run the risk of causing irreparable harm to your body. Eating when stressed doesn't have to be a bad thing. The key is to make sure you eat snacks that will enhance your body's performance.

Food is one of life's great treasures. It is meant to be enjoyed and shared. Despite this, it is important that we make our choices about what we eat and when we eat it. No longer can you be driven by pleasure, social comfort or stress relief. Eating is not wrong it is only when we eat for the wrong reason that damage takes place.

# CHAPTER 3


## *DIETING FOR LIFE. ONE DIET AFTER ANOTHER*

Diets by their very nature tend to be temporary. So how can we find one that we can live with day after day? Before we try to answer this question, let's take a look at some popular diets out there today.

South Beach:

The South Beach diet was developed by Florida based cardiologist Arthur Agatston, who prescribed this diet to his cardiac patients. The key points of the South beach diet are:

- Avoid consuming bad (i.e. simple) carbohydrates like sugar, sweets, white bread etc.

- Avoid fats that are bad for you (saturated fats, trans fats)

- Use a three-phased approach that aims at losing weight in the first phase and gradually introducing more variety as you move into phase three.

This diet is a fairly good one, although it may not be the most effective for weight loss. It also allows us to eat consume some foods that could be bad for us in the long run.

Atkins

Here is another very popular diet. This diet follows a low carbohydrate -high protein based regime. The diet uses the concept of ketosis; in which the body burns excess fat is burned as fuel, resulting in a loss in weight. Although this is an effective diet for weight reduction, it cannot be recommended as the 'best diet for life'.

A lot of people following the diet consume too much protein and excess fat, The diet does not emphasize the importance of fresh fruit and vegetables to our overall well-being. It should not be adopted as the best diet for life.

Sonoma Diet

This is another diet that uses a three phased approach to losing weight. Unlike the South Beach diet, it does allow the consumption of (whole grain) cereals and bread during the first phase. This is a very balanced diet. It is not as restrictive as many others and allows the individual more choice. Overall it is quite a good diet to follow in the long term.

Zone Diet

The Zone Diet was developed by biochemist Dr Barry Sears. He recommends that we get 40% of our calories from carbohydrates, 30% from protein and 30% from fat - unsaturated where possible.

This is a fairly balanced diet, and can be adopted on a daily basis. The drawback is the need to be conscious of the quantities we consume of each of the food groups. As an athlete I have followed this diet (approximately, without counting calories.) with good results.

The above are just a few of the many dieting programs available today. Which one will work best for you really depends on your needs today. Are you looking for a way to lose weight now, or just to maintain your current weight? The best diet is one that:

- meets your current weight loss needs

- you can live with on a daily basis

- is healthy and provides your body with the nutrients needed

- allows you to cheat occasionally

- includes an exercise program

Importance of Exercise

Many diet programs (especially those using weight loss pills) don't stress the need to exercise regularly. If you don't burn the same, or more, calories than you consume, then you'll never maintain your ideal weight. Walking, jogging, cycling and aerobics are all pleasurable exercises that will burn calories and contribute to your overall feeling of well-being.

The fact is, no one diet will probably do everything you need and you should review them all. If you want to lose weight then the Atkins diet is probably the most effective. Once you have lost the weight however, you need to select a regime that meets all the other criteria above.

The Sonoma diet is good, and so is the Zone. As long as you follow the basic guidelines, avoid junk food as much as possible and make sure you are getting a good intake of natural organic foods then you have probably found the best diet for your life.

A common misconception is that there is a best diet out there for everyone, that through some tweak we can make everyone live longer and achieve maximum physical condition by feeding them the perfectly optimized diet.

I imagine this as the food bar of the future that is closely related to meal bar often served in prison. This may be somewhat of an iron curtain type view but it is fueled by numerous people trying to determine what they need to eat to lose weight but still not taking action.

My simple answer is that diet depends. There are countless factors that go into choosing a healthy diet that maximizes a person's genetic profile and yes people respond to the same diet differently because of their particular genetic makeup.

It is asonine to think that everyone can thrive on a fast food standard American diet. It is not the least bit surprising that we are plagued by health problems that can be easily solved by diet.

Enough about simple genetics. Here are a couple more generalizations. Old and young populations requires significantly different diets. Heavily active individuals require more calories than their sedentary counterparts. People attempting to add or gain weight can have extreme diet differences. People recovering from sickness or disease have special requirements.

When selecting a healthy diet for yourself and yes you should give this some thought and forward planning in order to maximize health benefits.

You should first consider genetics and family history, the genetics part is a little more difficult but family history usually gives some pretty good clues about things that you may want to steer away from. Next you need to evaluate your lifestyle.

If you are a highly active person don't try a high deficit diet, you will be setting yourself up for failure and heart ache. Small simple changes are the easiest to implement and the most likely to stick.

Last, consider your goals, what body are you trying t achieve? The answers to these questions should give you a clear picture of how to proceed and how to structure your diet program.

Don't be afraid to make changes and add and subtract things from your diet. Variety is an excellent way to add different nutrients to your diet and find new and exciting flavors. Be adventurous and enjoy trying new things and learning how to maximize your physical and metal potential through one of the most simple bodily requirement

Many people often fail when it comes to dieting simply because of a poor choice of diet. They go for the low calorie diet where you don't eat, which is terrible for you. Or perhaps they go for the specialty diet, where they eat one type of food, or eat all types of food with the exception of a certain group.

There is nothing more dangerous than restricting your body from calories and all the major food groups. It is proven that your body needs certain types of food to function, so why would it make sense to remove one of these groups? It certainly doesn't.

The metabolism is easily set into a routine if you consistently eat the same food. When it is stuck in this routine it begins to slow down and after a while, it would lose a race against a snail.

## Yo-Yo Dieting

Yoyo Dieting is the main reason why majority of people are frustrated at their weight loss result. Having a well-toned, slim body has been the main concern for everybody especially before any special event. Everybody is always excited at any new opportunity to have a sexy body, to have a body that every one of our friends will envy.

This makes us buy almost anything that says we can achieve weight loss within minutes literally, only to get depressed at the result we get. we tend to lose weight, but only to regain it within a couple of months. Then we lose confidence in ourselves in our ability to lose weight, our excitement dampens, and we suffer from low self-esteem as a result.

Maybe this sounds like what you have been going through, well I must tell you that the major reason for this type of weight loss result is yoyo dieting. Most of the diet programs that are in circulation on the internet that promises a tremendous amount of weight loss within days are crash diets.

And because of our impatience (maybe you think that you have to lose weight before an event), we rush to buy such diet programs. You lose weight within this short period as promised, but only to regain it back within a couple of months.

Why do this happen?

Well let me take time to explain. Some diet programs are just too deterring, they take quality foods of your table. You cannot do this for such a long time before your body starts telling you that it is in need of quality diets. You go back to your old eating habits, this time at an alarming rate, which results in you gaining weight.

Also, most of these diet programs are crash diets. Your body needs nutrients to function. Such programs usually hide under the fact that you need calorie deficit (which you do anyway) to lose weight and therefore, you have to limit the intake of food so that your body can utilize more energy than it is given.

Yeah this is true, but the fact is that you have to know you daily calorie maintenance level; it is an important number if you are really serious about losing weight.

To avoid yoyo dieting, the amount of calories you need to take daily is this number less 500, anything less than that will not only starve you but also make you crave for extra calories, which results in those pounds that you have already lost to come back.

One of the things you must do is that you have to change the way you see weight loss, it is usually not as fast as you are made to believe. Yoyo dieting usually comes along when we think we can lose some certain amount of pounds before one special event; we crash diet.

But we know what comes next; we regain the weight that we have lost only to find it difficult to lose. Wouldn't you like to see weight loss as something that has to do with your lifestyle. Change your lifestyle for permanent weight loss, not because of a special occasion.

Talking about a total lifestyle change, see exercise as something you have to get involved with. You can't achieve weight loss without exercises, strength training to be precise. Seeing starvation as the only way that you can achieve you weight loss will only get you involved in yoyo dieting.

_Fad Diets: Single Food, Restrict Macro-Nutrient (i.e; Carbs, Fats etc.)_

Although the big push for fad diets has died down a little bit, it is still estimated that at least two-thirds of Americans are on some type of diet at any given time.

Although research shows the importance of eating from all the major food groups, people are still confused about what type of diet to follow, keeping the window open for more quickie solutions to pop up.

In an effort to help readers determine what makes a diet healthy and when it's time to steer clear, I am going to discuss what makes a diet a 'fad' diet and why these diets are something best to stay away from. Along the way, we will discover what each food group has to offer that can be beneficial to our health.

Our bodies are uniquely designed to take advantage of the proteins, carbohydrates and fats that we eat. In order for the liver to do the best job it can for us, we actually need all of these nutrients, known as macronutrients. Even a 'detoxifying' diet should also include all of these macronutrients.

Identifying a fad diet

A 'fad diet' is defined as something temporary. Therefore, it's no surprise that these diets are not successful. Let's begin by looking at how to identify a fad diet.

1 - Promises a fast weight loss.

This is great, in the short term, but how many readers have or know someone who has followed one of these diets, only to regain the weight back, plus more for added bonus?

When people lose weight very quickly, they lose a lot of lean muscle tissue, and the weight that comes back will most likely be more fat and less muscle, making it easier and easier to regain weight each time they drop the last fad diet.

A healthy diet to follow will be one that will encourage slow, progressive weight loss over a longer period of time. It will have enough calories to support vigorous exercise, so that you lose fat and not muscle.

Diets that are too low for the body's basic needs will result in the body breaking down it's protein stores (muscle) for the fuel it needs. Sort of defeats the whole purpose of the diet.

2 - Eliminates foods or food groups.

The very first thing that alerts us that a diet is a 'fad' is when a food, or entire food group, is considered off-limits. This is a good time to talk about the low carb diets.

What is it that has made carbohydrates a bad nutrient? When you look at other countries, where the intake of carbohydrates is as high as 80%, and see that many of these countries are not suffering even close to the obesity rates we are in America, you have to wonder why they are not having the same problem. So, can it really be the carbs?

Probably not. But, maybe it's the type of carbs. Many people who decide to go on one of the popular low carbohydrate diets start to eliminate a lot of food from their diets, including all the snack foods they were eating, particularly at night.

Gone are the chips, the cookies, the crackers, the ice cream. Gone are up to 300 to 1,000 calories per day. Anyone would lose weight if they cut out those many calories from their daily diet.

Another problem with eliminating entire food groups, especially on low carb diets, is that they are recommending eliminating or limiting the intake of nutrient-rich fruits and vegetables.

With all the substantial research showing how beneficial these foods are to preventing various diseases, such as cancer and heart disease, it's amazing that anyone involved in healthcare would recommend such a diet.

Something to also notice, however, is that none of these fad diet books are written by anyone with a degree in nutrition. Even the medical community is confused, which explains why physicians will fall for some of the hype fad diet authors write.

But let's talk a little more about fruits, vegetables and starches: A diet high in animal protein and animal fat has been linked to various disease and inflammation states. A diet very high in protein puts a great load on our kidneys and can contribute to constipation, gout and bone loss due to calcium depletion from the high protein load.

Combine that with decreased fiber from lack of whole grains and fiber-rich fruit and vegetables, and many people just don't feel well; they feel fatigued, sluggish and their immune system is depressed.

3 - Starts with a shock or follows a strict plan.

When the diet says you have to start with an extremely restricted diet, or you can only eat certain foods on particular days, you know it's a fad diet. They justify this by saying you have to clean out the body, or only certain foods will help with the weight loss process. Any change in how you currently eat will result in changes on the scale.

Very few people can remain on these diets very long, so once they are 'off' the diet, the weight returns. The dieter learned nothing other than the misinformation the author provided them with. This can have far-reaching consequences, as then the dieter is more confused than ever and doesn't know what to believe.

Once a person learns what the qualities of a healthy diet consist of, they find that their optimum calorie level is for their own needs, and they are able to achieve their goals, combining their eating plan with exercise. Not only do they start to enjoy life again, but enjoy food AND see weight loss.

Although fad diet authors want you to believe their 'miracle' (and buy their products), there really is no get-thin-quick solution that is permanent.

But what does constitute a healthy diet? A healthy diet is one that is adequate in calories to support healthy weight, low in animal fats and saturated fats, animal protein should be very lean and adequate enough to support a diet high in fruits and vegetables and whole grain starches.

Any healthy diet can include foods that are just for enjoyment, however. All foods really do fit, in moderation. A general rule is an 80/20 rule: Eighty percent of the time the diet should be healthy and then 20% of the time it can include foods you would not eat on a regular basis if you were trying to eat for health and weight loss.

4 - Contradicts what experts say.

Authors of low carb diets say that the carbohydrates are what have made American's fat. But they can't explain why other countries whose diets are very high in carbohydrates don't have the same problems with obesity.

You know it's a fad diet when the author says they have the 'inside' or 'hidden' truth about our health or diets. You also know it's a questionable publication when they say there is a hidden agenda among health professionals or the government.

5 - Relies on testimonials rather than scientific research.

The fact that Jane lost pounds in a week because she just ate cabbage soup does not mean it's safe, effective, or that it will work for you. What if you don't LIKE cabbage?

An example of testimonials, combined with the research to back it up, is the National Weight Control Registry. In order to join the Registry, a person must have lost pounds and have kept it off for a year.

Currently consisting of over 4500 individuals, the Registry was founded in 1993 as a longitudinal prospective study. Currently, there have been six studies resulting out of the Registry.

6 - Has a gimmick.

The problem with diet plans that have some type of gimmick, is people can't stay on them and they don't learn how to eat for the long-term. It's no secret that all the books must have something to 'catch' the reader.

However, hidden among all the hype are books that really DO offer safe and effective solutions to weight loss. A book written by a registered dietitian (RD) is a guarantee that the material is accurate and safe. An RD is someone whose education, training and experience all revolve around the science and practice of nutrition; these truly ARE nutrition experts.

## *Ways to Assure an Easy Diet For Life*

Uncovering an easy diet program in the myriad of choices today necessitates one scrutinize the character of each plan. Don't start any diet plan or weight loss program before you can spot the 5 obvious warning signs.

Now, without a doubt, I'd be willing to bet you've tried already, if not one, perhaps several diets before, AND, you've dropped weight and gained it all back, plus some, on all of them. It's that sort of disenchantment that tends to keep most of us from wanting to try ever again.

There is a simple explanation why it didn't work before. Apparently you were motivated and wanted to be healthy. But, it was not to be because you were required to take on a program of limited and fixed scope into and onto your body. It just doesn't work that way. You didn't even know that your failure wasn't your fault. You didn't know you were set up for failure.

You can correct those bad habits pretty easily, if you're truly motivated, and follow healthy diets for life. Making healthier food choices, eating at regular times of day and staying hydrated are just a few of the weight loss tips you'll find included below.

• Don't skip breakfast. Start your day right by giving your body the fuel it needs to produce energy throughout the day, and you won't suffer that mid-morning crash or slump and automatically reach for a pastry or another high calorie, zero nutrition, fat creating food.

Some excellent breakfast choices include oatmeal; eggs; fruits and whole grain breads, these should always be included in your diets for life.

• Take your time when eating, making sure you thoroughly chew your food, There are a number of good reasons to cultivate this habit. The stomach requires a minimum of 15 minutes to send the signal to the brain that it's full.

Eating slowly aids your digestive system in doing its job more easily, without necessitating the creation of large amounts of acid and other enzymes that break down larger food bits.

• Stay hydrated. Drinking ample amounts of good water daily is a key to good health and weight loss. Recent scientific research has proven what feels like a hunger pang or craving may be your body telling you it's dehydrated.

So be sure to drink several bottles or glasses of good water daily, as part of your diet for life - particularly when you feel a craving. You may find that a lot of them simply disappear.

• Try eating six small meals throughout the day rather than three larger ones. Choose healthy foods - fruits and proteins are both good for promoting healthy weight loss.

• Make sure your meals are rich in green leafy vegetables, beans, dark yellow fruits and vegetables.

• Eat only when you're truly HUNGRY and not just bored or trying to satiate an emotional need, rather than a true physical one. Include iron-rich foods in your diet, as iron deficiency can lead to problems such as anemia.

• Become a Label Reader. Take responsibility for what you're putting into your body. In this age of so many convenient pre-cooked microwaveable meals, if the label has more unpronounceable chemicals and preservatives than it does true food substances, those are things your digestive system doesn't know how to break down or have use for, and should never be incorporated in your diet for life. Simple and natural is always the healthiest, smartest choice.

• Avoid sodium and salt. These are notorious for causing high blood pressure and water weight retention. So steering clear of sodas (even diet ones) and highly salted foods is a great idea.

# CHAPTER 4

## *WHAT SHOULD YOU EAT?*

It is common knowledge that healthy eating and fitness of the body is the secret to good health and longevity. But, due to our hectic lifestyles, we often ignore this simple truth and end up feeling tired with hardly any energy to make it through the day.

But if you truly wish to change this bad situation for the better, there is hope. There are a number of ways in which you can fit healthy eating in your busy schedule and undo years of self-indulgence.

An unbalanced diet or one deficient in essential nutrients will make you feel weak, lethargic and reduce your performance to below par. Healthy eating and fitness go hand-in-hand. Nutritionists will tell you that you must eat right to look and feel healthy as well as have the energy to lead an active lifestyle.

They will also tell you that a portion control diet is the key to reclaiming your health and to do this you must eat a variety of foods from the different food groups. Your daily diet should include vegetables, fruits, whole grains, milk and dairy products, meats, poultry and eggs.

Fitness depends on healthy eating and daily food planning to get the right nutritional value from your food. You must follow a diet that is rich in fiber. Select foods that have high fiber content like fruits, vegetables and whole grains.

Your diet should also be low in saturated fats and cholesterol, so go easy on the cheese, butter and margarine. Instead, choose dairy products and use unsaturated fats like olive and canola oil in your cooking. Meats are a great source of protein but ensure that you eat lean meats so that you don't over consume unwanted fats.

Healthy eating is what fitness is all about and your daily trips to the fast food joint would obviously have to happen no more than once a month. Food from restaurants and takeaways is high in sodium, saturated fats and low in fiber - not a healthy diet if you wish to keep fit.

Healthy eating also means limiting your sodium and sugar intake as well as taking alcoholic drinks in moderation. Above all, drink plenty of water (at least 8 glasses a day) to keep your body hydrated. Water also helps to move the nutrients throughout your body and flush out the toxins.

The first step to daily healthy eating plans involves a change in food as well as eating behavior. Don't skip meals - eat three large meals and a couple of mini meals each day. Most of us tend to skip breakfast which is the most important meal of the day. Remember our moms told us so.

A good healthy eating breakfast increases the metabolism and gives you the energy to start off your day. Also, eating a series of meals through the day ensures that your stomach is not empty, thus preventing you from overeating at meal time.

Observing serving sizes of food is necessary. Watch those portions or better still, use portion control plates and scoopers to make it easier to get the right amount of essential nutrients the body needs.

Healthy eating should be balanced with exercise to achieve fitness of the body as well as the mind. Making a conscious effort to eat healthy foods for a healthy diet and being disciplined enough to exercise at least twice or thrice a week will help with your fitness program as well as your weight management program.

## *All Natural, High Fiber Foods To Eat for 25 Grams of Daily Recommended Fiber*

If you know anything about health and fitness then you know 25 grams of fiber are recommended daily for a healthy, balanced diet. However, do you know which foods are high enough in fiber to help you reach that level every day? Here are 5 simple resources to keep in mind when selecting foods for 25 grams of fiber in your day.

1. "An apple a day keeps the doctor away". Fuji, Gala, Golden Delicious Pink Lady, Granny Smith and McIntosh apples each provide 5 grams of fiber.

Apples are quite possibly, the easiest, high fiber foods to eat. There are many varieties to choose from, and in a few minutes you can quickly pick up 5 grams of fiber. The choices are plenty, they're relatively inexpensive and apples provide a perfect source of nutritional fiber in a convenient, ready to eat package.

No cooking or preparation required, except for a little rinsing. You can eat them on the go, in the car, at work, or even in bed. Of course we all have heard, "An apple a day keeps the doctor away".

2. Black beans provide as much as 7g of fiber per 1/4 cup of dry beans. 1/4 cup of Pinto Beans rings up a hefty 12g of fiber per

serving and Garbanzo Beans are the tops with 9g of fiber per 1/4 cup serving.

Yes, it's true beans are good for your heart and they are really good food to eat for their high fiber content. Very few foods with as much nutrition are as versatile, economical and flavorful as beans. There are many ways to prepare beans or to order them while dining out.

Soups often provide a good source of beans. You may even enjoy a few beans in a salad, or try the ever popular, rice and beans. Fast food chains sometimes have bean burritos, bean chili, or salads with beans on the menu.

3. "Breakfast is the most important meal". A bowl of shredded wheat, a piece of toast with multi grain bread, or an all bran muffin are wholesome high fiber food choices for breakfast. Each one can give you 3-5g of fiber or more and they are easy to prepare.

It may or may not be the most important meal, but breakfast is usually the first opportunity to start your day with plenty of fiber. Orange juice and apple juice even go nicely with an all-bran muffin for added fiber first thing in the morning.

4. "Shake it up and go". Get 5g of fiber in a cold, delicious chocolate or strawberry shake.

Now, it's easy to find, on the Internet, some high quality health drinks that provide excellent sources of soluble fiber. In fact, one high fiber protein drink even provides FOS, fructooligasacharides, a pro-biotic soluble fiber that is typically found in foods like onion, garlic, oats, and barley.

High fiber health drinks make it easy to mix up a delicious shake with a few pieces of frozen banana or other fruit, for a cold, creamy, tasty way to start the day with 5g of fiber.

5. "High fiber food is good for your mood". A high fiber food bar should give you at least 4g of fiber in a serving. If it doesn't, then it isn't worth the calories.

When you eat plenty of fiber you feel better. Try a high fiber food bar for a quick snack any time of day and feel good about yourself without the guilt of snacking on junk food. People eat candy bars, power bars, and all kinds of bars that offer little or no fiber.

### What Should I Eat For Muscle Building?

People are always looking for the best muscle building foods, or foods that will help them pack on the most amount of muscle. I always suggest eating a wide and varied diet that includes the three macronutrients i.e. protein, carbs and fats.

Top this off with the micronutrients of vitamins and minerals and you have a decent diet. So where do you get these nutrients? The following will help you find out the best foods to consume.

Proteins

Everyone knows that protein is crucial for muscle building and head straight for the supplements. However you can get plenty of protein from your daily diet. Meat, fish and poultry provide many different sources for getting enough protein.

Any kind of meat such as beef, chicken, lamb, duck are good as long as you go for the leanest cuts of meat. Any seafood is also excellent and brings many other health benefits such as healthy oils and high Omega-3 and Omega-6 levels. In a muscle building diet you should get about 40% of your calories from protein.

Carbs

One of the most misunderstood macronutrients in the health and fitness world is carbs. Carbs are actually a crucial part of any bodybuilding diet plan. Carbs are essential for energy throughout your day and especially your workouts.

When you begin your workout and your energy stores are not full your body will begin to use vital protein for energy. This is protein you want to keep for muscle building. So therefore eat carbs with your meals throughout the day. On a muscle building diet about 45% of your calories should come from carbs.

Where should you get these carbs? You are going to need to eat complex carbs. These are slow releasing and stop you from getting insulin spikes. No good when controlling your diet. You can obtain complex carbs from sources such as wholemeal pasta, brown rice, brown bread, and many vegetables.

Fats

Another misunderstood macronutrient that is needed in your diet is fats. Most people think that fat makes you fat. However, the truth is if you eat more calories than you burn off you will gain weight. In muscle building you will want to over eat in order to grow but don't shun the fats.

Fats enable your body to digest vital fat soluble vitamins A, D, E and K. As your body needs these to grow, you should get at least 15% of your calories from fats. You can obtain these from olive oil, nuts and seeds.

Fruit and veg

Fruit and veg is a great way to get complex and simple carbs into your diet. They also bring a whole host of health benefits to your body. This is what will boost muscle growth. By having a wide and varied diet that provides everything your body needs then it will grow and grow fast. Any fruit or veg is good for your diet. However, the top ones would be spinach, broccoli, cabbage, apples and oranges and bananas.

Water

One of the most important components to your diet is water. Water makes up a large portion of your body and is responsible for most of the processes that go on in your body. Therefore water is crucial to muscle growth, uptake of protein and all the nutrients you needs

Therefore there are a large variety of muscle building foods that will help you build muscle. The best thing is to ensure you eat a varied diet to make sure your body gets everything it needs to grow muscle.

## *Foods to Eat For Strength Training*

Your fitness training routine will include exercises that you have put together after much thought. However, you need to put an equal amount of thought into what you are eating for an all-rounded fitness-training schedule.

If you are undertaking strength-training exercises, protein is one nutrient you should include in abundance in your meals for muscle recovery. You need to choose high-quality protein and take it at appropriate times. It works along with carbohydrates and fats to keep your body working at its best.

You should have regular protein dosages throughout the day, especially after your workouts. Getting protein after strength training will restore muscle tissue that has been stressed during the workout.

I have put together a list of power foods that will provide you your required protein. These foods in most cases can even fulfill your protein needs without turning to supplements. As it is, nutritional experts say your body benefits more from a well-rounded wholesome diet plan than supplements.

1. Lean Beef

This is an ideal source of protein. You can include it in your meals in stir-fried form. A combo of lean beef with rice and vegetables makes for a scrumptious meal which is rich in carbohydrates, fiber and protein. This meal is perfect to have after workouts. 20-30 grams of this meal after exercise, is enough.

2. Eggs and egg whites

Eggs are one of the highest-quality protein sources available. They have all the necessary amino acids you need for healthy muscles.

An omelet with summer vegetables along with whole-grain toast gives you 25 grams of protein and 15% of your daily fiber needs. For those of you who are keeping a watch on your cholesterol intake, you can use egg whites in this recipe or egg substitutes.

3. Protein-rich soy

Use tofu to make a filling and tasty burger. This cholesterol-free protein source is good for your heart and muscles. A Grilled Lemon-Basil Tofu Burger will give you 10.5 grams of protein. Peppery watercress and fresh tomatoes will give you additional nutrients of Vitamins A and C.

4. White Grains with Protein

Quinoa has higher protein content than most whole grains. It is a mild grain with a chewy texture. Cooking it in broth lends it even more flavor. A Black Bean-Quinoa Salad is made more delicious with black beans, lima beans and tofu. Drizzle it with Basil-lemon dressing. This vegetarian salad has about 10 grams of protein per serving.

No doubt you want to eat for health and fitness, but many people today have the idea that they can't because of the cost.

Well, although food prices are definitely on the rise these days, it's still possible for you to eat good foods for fitness without breaking the bank. Here are some important tips that can help you to eat healthy foods without having to spend a huge amount of money.

Never Shop When You're Hungry

One of the most important tips that can really help you save and insure that you eat right is to never shop when you are hungry. When you go shopping while hungry, it's a recipe for disaster.

You'll end up making bad food decisions based on your hunger and you'll just about always end up spending more money in the grocery store. So, before you go out to brave the grocery store, eat something so you are not hungry. This will definitely help you save money and you'll avoid bringing home unhealthy foods too.

## Purchase Foods that are Generic

If you are looking for healthy foods but you don't want to spend a fortune eating for fitness, consider purchasing foods that are generic. Many people think that generic brands are inferior, but usually you'll find that the food's nutritional value is no different than the name brand. Purchasing a generic brand of foods can save you a bundle on healthy foods.

## Shop the Sales on Healthy Foods

Shopping the sales on health foods is another great tip that can help you to eat for fitness without breaking the bank. Many stores offer sales and you can save quite a bit of money if you follow those sales.

Look in the Sunday paper or for grocery store ads that you receive in the mail. You'll be able to find out where the best deals are on the healthy foods that you want to purchase.

## Portion Out Healthy Snacks Yourself

Today stores are making big money on healthy snacks that are already portioned out. Often you will find them in servings of 100 calories. While having portioned snacks is definitely a great idea for your health, buying them this way can cost quite a bit.

You can save a lot of money by purchasing larger portions of food items and portioning out healthy snack portions yourself. Purchase a box of re-sealable baggies and bag up your own snacks. This way the snacks are quick for you to grab and you won't overeat.

Purchase Water Instead of Other Drink Options

There are many drink options available when you go shopping. Sadly, most of them are bad for you. Avoid purchasing sports drink, high calories juices, and sodas. If you do decide you want juice, make sure that there is not sugar added to the juice.

The better choice is to purchase water instead. Water is much better for you, it will improve your health, and you'll also find that it is cheaper to purchase than the other unhealthy drinks.

These are just a few of the ways that you can eat for fitness while saving money. You won't break the bank and the whole family will be eating healthy. It's easy to do and you'll still feel happy with the foods you have in the home.

Eating right is an important element of bodybuilding success, especially if you're a beginning athlete.

Sound nutrition will help you maintain a steady level of energy and ensure you can complete each and every workout session; the only way you'll be able to build muscle and strength in the long-term is by eating enough calories throughout the day and getting enough rest.

Eating the wrong foods at the wrong time can set you up for disaster, and severely limit your performance and muscle gains.

# CHAPTER 5

## *AVERAGE FITNESS IS BETTER THAN TOO MUCH OR TOO LITTLE FITNESS*

Let's say your exercise of choice is running. Maybe you can only manage to run a few minutes before your heart feels like it's about to explode out of your chest and you're forced to stop for fear of passing out. It's going to take you a while to build up to 30 minutes if you simply run your maximum each day and then stop.

So instead of that, try running 1 minute then walking 1 minute, repeating this cycle for as long as you can. You'll find that you can go much further without overtaxing your heart and muscles. Maybe you can even go 10-20 minutes your first time.

If run 1 walk 1 is too hard, try run 1 walk 2 or run 2 walk 3. Experiment to see what intervals work best for you. If your heart is still racing after the walking interval, increase the walking interval and/or reduce the running interval.

I recommend you aim for an initial interval that allows you to do the most amount of running in a 25 minute period. If you can only manage run 1 walk 4, that's fine.

Take a week to experiment with different intervals if you need to, but find one that allows you to go 25 minutes total (even if it's run 1 walk 24). You should be physically challenged but not to the point of feeling nauseous or faint.

Once you're able to go 25 minutes, gradually increase the running time and reduce the walking time. Aim to reach run

1 walk 1 for 25 minutes for an initial goal. Be patient as it may take you a few weeks to get there if you're starting with a longer walking interval.

Next, gradually increase the running period while keeping the walking period at 1 minute. Go from run 1 walk 1 to run 1:30 walk 1. Then try run 2 walk 1. Keep extending your running intervals until you can manage run 8 walk 1 for 25 minutes.

Now keep those intervals the same, and gradually build your time from 25 minutes to 45 minutes. Don't worry about distance, and don't be concerned if you run a little slower. Just put in the time. Aim to increase the total time by about 10% per week, which roughly averages out to adding about 30 seconds per day.

Once you can do run 8 walk 1 for 45 minutes, you can switch to running continuously. You'll likely find you're able to do 25 minutes continuously without any trouble. After that you can continue to increase the distance, build your speed, do harder forms of interval training, or just maintain your current routine.

The advantage of this type of interval training is that you're still spending most of the time in your aerobic range, so your circulatory system will get the benefit of that conditioning.

If you're out of shape, the running intervals will spike your heart rate quickly, and your heart rate will take a while to come back down, so even while walking you'll still be mostly in the aerobic range.

But you'll avoid burning out from having your heart rate get too high. Walking won't tire your muscles as much as running, so your legs won't give out as quickly, and you won't be quite as sore after your runs.

You can adapt this idea to other aerobic exercises as well. For swimming you can switch to a slower stroke or a glide. For bike riding you can coast instead of pedal hard.

This technique is also useful for distance running. Some people run marathons in a pattern of run 7 walk 1 (or similar intervals), and they often find their finishing times are better vs. when they run continuously. The brief walking periods slow you down in the early miles, but they make up for it in later miles by keeping your running muscles fresh.

So you end up maintaining an even pace even through those last 6 miles where many people hit the wall. I once used a run 7 walk 1 pattern for a 13-mile training run, and I finished in 2 hours, which was a good time for me. I felt I was running strong all the way without dragging at the end.

Even if you're terribly out of shape, you can use mild interval training to rebuild your fitness to a healthy level without causing yourself tremendous pain and discomfort. And it probably won't take that long.

A typical marathon training program can take you from running 3 miles to running 26.2 miles in six months, and that requires much more time and effort than going from 0 to 3 miles.

From how heavy you are and how much weight you want to lose, to your allergies, your current diet and how flexible you can be about changing it, and, of course, how active you currently are, you must consider the best health and exercise plan for you.

So there are certainly a handful of variables to take into account which are specific to the person who wants to lose weight and stay healthy.

The numbers of calories you consume per day is very important to take into consideration, especially when you are altering your diet to loose or maintain a certain wait.

The thing that most people do not understand is that sometimes calorie count can be crucial for your success. Many people actually have no idea how many calories they consume per day. Often, you will find that specific food items contain a lot more calories than you would think.

Nonetheless, to keep track of your calorie intake it is a simple thing to do when you go by the information on the labels of virtually all grocery store food items. It is a bit harder to do if you are eating fast food and / or junk food.

The latest scientific research has discovered the following estimates: instead of the suggested 2,000 calories per day on which daily value percentages are based, most people (or in total average people) is 2,195. Fifty percent of that amount is estimated to be carbohydrates, thirty-four percent (again, average) calories from fat, fifteen percent accounted for is protein, and two percent of the calories accounted for are from alcohol.

It has been strongly recommend by doctors, nutritionists, and other professionals that women require an average of 1600 to 2000 calories per day if they want to maintain their weight.

To lose weight, however, it is recommended that women eat between 1200 and 1600 calories. Nonetheless, depending on the average amount of calories that you already take in per day, you may want to reduce your calorie intake more slowly.

You can use a calorie counter as a piece of weight loss equipment, these little gadgets will be able to approximate how many calories you burn as you exercise. It will also count calories you burn while you do various activities.

The basic performance of a calorie counter is a technological process that considers your daily activities, as well as the amount of intensity of those activities, (for example: a one hour walk verses a one hour workout class) and, of course, your current weight. With this information, the device keeps track of all the calories you have burned.

To get an idea of the differences in calories burned between different kinds of exercises such as walking, swimming, etc. it also depends on your weight. For example: one hour of basic, easy exercises such as walking will burn approximately two hundred and seventy calories if the individual is around one hundred and fifty pounds.

This is significantly less than the calories that he or she will burn doing something like playing basketball for an hour (for someone of about the same weight, of course) which will burn almost five hundred and thirty calories.

There are a few tips I can give you to start lowering the number of calories and fats you consume per day. Try taking in less sugar, cooking oils, eat foods high in fiber, do not fry foods, grill them or boil them instead, and most importantly, consult a dietician who can help you plan meals for yourself.

As a matter of fact, there are even some fruits and vegetables that contain what are referred to as negative calories, these will, in fact, help you burn off calories effortlessly. Among these fruits and vegetables are melons, strawberries, peaches, grapefruit, cauliflower, cucumber, broccoli, lettuce, beans and celery. I have even heard it said that chewing a bite of some of these green vegetables, such as celery, burns more calories than the amount of calories in the bite itself. Ergo, negative calories.

Another thing to really watch for if you are trying to lose weight, maintain your current weight, or just eat healthier foods, is your fat intake. Fats are the cells that develop and fill your lipids.

Liposuction comes from the word lipid, and the procedure actually removes the lipids from your body, whereas when you lose weight, you simply remove the fats from the lipids in your body. There are three different kinds of fats, saturated fats, unsaturated fats, and monounsaturated fats.

Certain daily activities can burn calories, for example: if you have a more active job or if you participate in sports, or even (as logic dictates) taking care of young children at home. However, many people sit behind a desk most of the day working.

To begin regular exercise at a slow pace, one of the first, most simple things you can do, no matter where you go, is to park far away from the entrance of the building.

Whether you are going to work, whether you are going to the grocery store, hardware store, movie theatre etc. when you park further you walk more. Walking is very important, especially for people just getting started and trying to build up to an even more fat - burning routine.

Another idea is to remember to take the stairs, as opposed to the elevator, in whatever building. These, among regularly walking at night or in the morning, are a good way to get started. Some people who have trouble setting up a regular walking routine have discovered that buying a dog is an incentive.

Dogs have to be walked, and often will run and want to be played with. Activities like this will burn calories and, while fun and loving, they will not feel like exercise, and will likely bring a big smile to your face. The more energy you have and the more active you become, you will notice that you just feel a lot better than before in the mind and in the body.

Fat intake will vary depending on the person. That is why you can follow general rules and see if they will help you, or you can visit a doctor or specialist in the field of nutrition who can help you. When you have the diet and exercise plan that works for you, you will be really happy, not only with how you look, but with how you feel.

You can play with your grandkids more, you can run and exercise and your energy and / or stamina will increase. You will not be held back by an unhealthy heart, lungs, or any other physical problems. And in addition, you will battle the blues, stress, or any bad thoughts in your mind because the brain is a vital organ that will be strengthened too.

Most of the most important kinds of fats are the unsaturated fats which are in oils such as vegetable oil. Monounsaturated fats are in virtually all oils and fatty foods. Lastly the least desirable are saturated fats. Usually a person should not consume more than thirty percent fat of the total calories from the foods he or she eats.

Saturated fat is the bad kind of fat (if you are concerned about fat intake) make sure that you pay extra attention to the amount of saturated verses unsaturated fats in the overall amount of fats you eat each day.

Remember, you should not cut fats out of your diet. Even if you did, any sugars will become fats if you eat too much. Your body needs a certain amount of fat to survive. Fats are what provide your body with maximum energy, and help retain vitamins.

There are essential fat soluble vitamins that go through the body as the fats are digested. In addition, of course, fats insulate the body and retain heat, this is why especially thin people become colder and heavier individuals are more likely to be warmer than others, on average.

Here come the details about exercise in the equation: there is no amount of diet change, or diet pills, or anything else that can replace the benefits of exercise. Without exercise, your body will retain instead of burning the amount of fats and carbohydrates you eat.

It has been said that someone should eat more than two hours but less than four hours before he or she exercises. However, I work out in the morning, therefore, I usually eat a piece of fruit or drink some milk or juice about a half an hour before I work out, and after I finish I will eat my full breakfast.

The most important thing about exercise is that it is the very best way to keep you healthy and will virtually always end up providing an individual with a longer, more exciting life.

No matter how you choose to exercise, whether you use gyms exercise equipment, home exercise equipment, home workout videos or anything else. Cardiovascular workouts are one of the most recommended kinds of workouts you can have.

Utilize the virtually endless types of exercises available for you on the market today. There are different kinds of home exercise equipment for virtually any space you have to work with, whether it is a home, an apartment or even a studio.

From aerobic, Pilates, yoga and other videos and / or DVDs, to elliptical exercise machines, treadmills, to yoga equipment and accessories such as balls and rubber bands etc. find what you prefer.

You can even take aerobic classes at the gym, find a personal trainer and/or small group fitness instructors and much, much more . . . you can find the perfect solution for you.

It has been estimated that the average individual will burn certain numbers of calories per hour depending on the kind of exercise they choose. For example: bicycling is said to burn about five hundred and forty five calories per hour.

Well, if you have ever taken a cycling class or two, or if you own your own indoor cycling exercise equipment, you know that that can vary significantly depending on how hard you push yourself.

Bicycling outdoors is the same, are you bicycling for an hour on rocky terrain, uphill or downhill or on a relatively flat path. The number of miles you ride in one hour is another of all of the variables to consider that can significantly change the number of calories you can burn on a bike.

The same applies with any kind of workout equipment, or favorite kinds of exercising such as running, for instance.

Running is a great way to workout but how many miles do you run in one hour? At what pace do you run? On what kind of trail or terrain do you run? There are people who stick to insisting on the average five hundred and forty five calories burned per hour for runners as well, but it is not so black and white.

There are easier activities which can be more accurately assessed to predict the number of calories burned. For example: bowling.

Because it is a very regular, timed activity (the only variables depending on a two player game verses a four player game, or a five player game etc.) it is much easier to calculate the number of calories burned playing, especially when you use the correct bowling technique.

I think that most importantly a person should decide based on the physical exercise they need and the kinds of exercise and / or exercise equipment he or she prefers, which exercise plan they will enjoy the most.

The perfect formula for success is a balance of exercise and diet, considering your calorie intake as well as your fat intake as I have explained above.

When you take the very best care of your body, you will not only look the very best you possibly can, but you will also feel your absolute best. You will be surprised at how much of a difference getting fit can make in your life.

### Cardio: Walking is better than running (joints) in the long run

You hear a lot of people talk about how running is bad for your knees, how it jars you around too much, and things like that. This leads a lot of people to believe that running is not good for you.

So, the next logical thing to ask is whether walking gives you the same benefits without the negative side effects? Is walking actually better than running? I would say there are pros and cons to each, depending on your goals. It has been my experience that it is good to do both.

Basically, you run for a set amount of time, then you walk for a set amount of time, and repeat that pattern throughout the race. I usually ran 7 minutes and walked 1 minute.

The key is to start the pattern right away, before you get tired. It feels a little weird at first switching to walking 7 minutes into a race while everyone else has their starting line energy boost.

People will be passing you like crazy. Just stay steady. Stick with the plan. They may be passing you at mile 1, but rest assured, your time will come at around mile 15. They'll be dropping back by the masses while you drift by like you just started the race.

Besides giving you a good advantage in marathons walking is just as beneficial for your fitness as running. Both are great for you if you develop proper form. I found a 2 hour seminar presented by a physical therapist on proper running form that really changed the way I run.

By understanding the mechanics of how the body reacts when it is running you can really conserve a lot of energy as well as prevent a lot of injuries. If you can find a similar class or seminar it would be well worth your time.

If you're just trying to stay fit, then walking is absolutely just as effective as running. If you really want to boost your endorphin level, I think running has a slight advantage. If you are competing in marathons or half marathons I really believe the run/walk method has a lot of advantages.

Of course, if you are an elite runner with marathon times below 3 hours you are probably going to lose time by doing a run/walk. However, if you're a mid-packer just trying to improve your personal best, then run/walk will work great for you.

Just remember this: When it comes to exercise moving is better than not moving. So, if you're not feelin' the run on a particular day, just walk.

## *Resistance training*

As you get older, you may experience different health problems such as a decreased metabolism, weight gain, blocked arteries, high blood pressure, diabetes, thinning of bones and accumulation of fat around belly and hips. Fortunately, fitness and cardio exercises make a wonderful way for elderly people to avoid these problems.

However, most of the seniors think that resistance training and fitness exercises are just for youngsters and they can't get benefit from the weight training exercises to gain muscle mass and a strong body.

This belief is just a myth and a recent research has revealed that resistance training and fitness exercises can greatly benefit elderly people even older than 60.

Weight training and cardiovascular exercises not only help the elderly to be healthy physically but psychologically as well. These exercises help them to tone their bodies and strengthen their muscles. Moreover, fitness exercises help the elderly to reduce their loneliness, stress and depression.

When elderly people go to the gym, they found a friendly and pleasant atmosphere over there, which helps to heighten their moods. They enjoy a healthy social life because they interact with their trainer and gym colleagues.

A recent study suggests that fitness and resistance training exercises can be very helpful in slowing down the aging process. Nearly all of the weight training and cardiovascular exercises enhance the intake of oxygen into your body.

This, in turn, allows your cells to absorb more oxygen and stay healthy. Moreover, cardiovascular exercises such as swimming, jogging, hiking, walking etc. keep your blood vessels and heart healthy, thus reducing the chances of sudden heart attack and other cardiovascular problems.

Weight training makes a great gift for elderly people because these exercises help them keep their blood pressure and blood sugar at appropriate levels. Diabetes Mellitus is a common problem among people who are over 50 years old.

Resistance training exercises help the elderly to burn their calories and utilize energy from their own bodies. Therefore, they can avoid potential threats of high blood pressure and diabetes by performing resistance training exercises.

Resistance training also helps seniors to lose body fat and maintain a healthy weight. It helps them to gain muscle mass, develop a strong and flexible body and build upper as well as lower body muscles. Other benefits of weight training for elderly people include a smooth blood flow, improved body balance, stronger bones and lubricated joints.

Resistance training offers many health benefits to the body. Resistance training's benefits to health include: muscles and bone strengthening, faster metabolism, fat burning, improvement of the cardiovascular system, and better overall health.

It increases the rate of metabolism which results In a body fat reduction. Resistance type of training, like weights lifting, is effective in burning more calories during the workout.

Furthermore, you will also boost your basal metabolism, which is the metabolism even after the workout. This results in more effective body fat reduction. Thus, you will notice two things: you lose the fat, making you leaner, and your body becomes firmer.

Because resistance training effectively boosts metabolism, this results in an overall increase in your fitness level. This will allow you to be able to handle more physical activities and lead an active lifestyle.

These types of exercises can also increase our overall strength due to a stronger and more powerful skeletal and muscular system. Weight lifting will strengthen the skeletal system, an important element which is critical as we age.

It likewise increases the bone mineral density. It can be helpful in maintaining bone health and minimizing the onset of bone maladies like osteoporosis.

Weight training can greatly improve cardiovascular health too. By strengthening the cardiovascular system, this can help lower our blood pressure and this is a good way to reduce the risk of heart diseases.

The question now is how to get started. Although most resistance training can only be done in the gym with weights, you can always exercise at home. Get a good Swiss ball and you can always get a good workout using your body weight as resistance such as isometric exercises.

Examples of these exercises are push-ups, ball squats, and Swiss bridges. You can always do these exercises at home at your own pace and enjoy the health benefits of resistance training.

## Combining Cardio & Resistance Training For Intense Workouts

Usually people who are into fitness exercise at least three times a week or exercise every other day either at gyms or other places where they can do their own workouts. Doing cardio and resistance training alternately produces a good foundation for good physical fitness. Not bad if you have the time, the problem is, most of us don›t.

So, instead of doing one type per session why not combine them both in a single session. This will give you maximum benefit per training. A simple example would be to do weights for about five to 10 repetitions then do some cardio like squat and run in place. After that, do the next bicep curls and do some jumping jacks, and so on for about forty minutes.

Do whatever exercise you feel like doing or for what areas you are targeting to tune up. Do major body part exercises as much as possible. Alternating on weights and thirty second cardio is a good routine. At least three sets alternating would be good enough for a fat burning calorie exercise.

What is being suggested here is not for those who are now getting started; this is a hard workout for beginners. Your breathing will become heavy and more intense. Don't do this if you have a weak heart or at least try to do it slowly at first. Just add more as you progress and when you have started to get the hang of it maybe after about a week or two.

The good thing about this is that it cuts down your workout time in half. Doing the three cycle sets is not easy at first. Don't push yourself to the limit, stop if you need to and catch your breath before trying to complete it. Improvement is gradual as it starts to be your regular routine.

## *Isometric Exercises - Some Common Questions Answered*

Isometric Exercises are a form of training in which the muscles attempt to contract and move but are prevented from doing so. So, curling a dumbell is not an isometric movement. However, trying to push against an immovable object like a house is an isometric contraction.

Often, this form of exercise is called self-resistance as one limb is often pitted against another. Isometrics have been around for thousands of years and are a major part of disciplines like Yoga and the Martial Arts.

They were a major part of the physical culture movement in both North America and Europe, but have died off somewhat during the second half of the last century. It is not my intention in this chapter to go into why this happened. Rather, I want to answer some common questions you might have about isometric exercises:

What is the concept of the isometric contraction and why is it so effective?

The whole point of performing an isometric contraction is to get to the last rep "first". Let me explain. Let's say you are performing some barbell curls. The whole point of weight lifting is to continue the movement until you cannot lift it anymore.

You are trying to train to the point of failure by exhausting all of the muscle fibers in your arm. When you perform an isometric exercise, you are attempting to do the same thing. Here's how it works.

Every muscle in your body is made up off different fibers that have varying levels of strength, explosiveness, and stamina. When you perform a fast motion like throwing a ball, you are utilizing the fast twitch muscles in your arm.

When you push against a heavy object, you are utilizing the slower twitch fibers. When you perform an isometric contraction, you are forcing ALL the fibers to become engaged.

Mother nature is very efficient. She always uses the exact minimum number of muscle fibers she has to for any movement. If she can get away with using two muscles to throw a ball, that's all she uses.

However, with isometrics, you are constantly straining, but NEVER moving. This forces your body to use every muscle fiber RIGHT away. This is the secret of isometric contractions, and why they allow you to «get to the last rep, first».

Can I get a complete workout using isometric exercises alone?

There are many components to fitness and being healthy. They are strength, flexibility, endurance (both muscular and cardio wise) balance, coordination, reaction time and aesthetics. Isometrics are very good at building strength and aesthetics.

It can also prepare you for other physical activities that will improve the other components I just mentioned. However, it will not dramatically improve them by itself.

Still, as a form of exercise that can be done quickly and will also improve your look and strength, they really can't be beat.

How long do I need to hold an isometric contraction to get the full effect?

This really depends on you and what you want to achieve. The more intense the contraction, the shorter it should be held for. An isometric contraction of 80% of your maximum should not be held longer than 12 seconds.

This is used for building maximum strength. However, if you want to build muscle size, you will want to hold the contraction at 35% of your max for 2 to 3 minutes. Of course, if you want to build size, you need to watch your diet as well.

Do isometric exercises pose the same risk of injury as other forms of strength training?

When performed correctly with proper breathing procedures, isometric training is probably the safest form of strength training that there is. There is no worries about lifting weights in an awkward fashion or straining yourself.

The key is to slowly build up the tension while breathing in for 4 seconds, holding the contraction for 7 seconds while your breathe out, then letting the tension dissipate while your breathe in again for 4 seconds.

# CHAPTER 6

MENTAL HEALTH

In the realm of the physical, it's universally recognized (albeit not always practiced), that if you want a healthy body, you've got to do preventative maintenance: brush your teeth, eat reasonably healthy food, exercise, get enough rest. Day in and day out we engage in a host of chores designed to help enhance the well-being and longevity of our physical selves.

In other words, we understand that physical fitness is a precursor to physical health. Yet, in matters pertaining to our mental and emotional selves, we find a different story.

Developing habits to nourish and exercise our mental and emotional selves is not something regularly considered by most Americans.

On the contrary, most of our effort aimed at attending to our mental and emotional needs are more about coddling than fitness. Feeling stressed? Grab a beer with friends. Sadness got you down? Go see the latest blockbuster movie. Anxious about work? How about a round of golf?

Rather than increasing our mental capacity, we medicate ourselves. We engage in activities to make us feel better in the short run, but without really addressing the root problem which revolves around an insufficient ability to absorb and cope with life's difficulties.

It's like addressing your weight gain by removing all the mirrors in the house. Sure it may make you temporarily feel better, but what does it do to solve the problem?

The truth is it's an approach that all too often produces what can only be described as free-range, feral minds.

Mental Fitness Defined

To be clear, in this context Mental Fitness does not refer to the development of knowledge or even mental acuity. This is an important point. Many of the mental activities we undertake to develop our minds have very little to do with Mental Fitness, as referred to here. Examples of activities that DON'T dramatically increase our Mental Fitness levels include:

Digesting data as part of the learning process

Exercising one's cognitive facility to make the mind more nimble

Participating in activities that soothe and nurture the agitated mind and emotions

This is not to say that these activities aren't worthy and valuable, for they obviously are vital in our development as productive and happy human beings.

Even so, for the most part, they are not helping to increase our ability to synthesize a relatively ease-filled experience in the most challenging of circumstances. And cultivating that ease-filled experience is the heart of Mental Fitness.

The key to the understanding of Mental Fitness is the notion of capacity. Mental Fitness is the measure of one's capacity to weather life's challenges without being thrown unduly off balance. It's the capacity to withstand a layoff, to bear a health diagnosis, or to endure a financial challenge with grace, and a sense of confident calm.

We all know people like this, who never seem to be ruffled. A layoff? No problem. IRS audit? Fine. A traffic accident? No biggie.

While everyone around them is sent into tailspins, these folks stay calm, cool, and collected no matter what life throws at them. So what is it about these people that makes them so well-equipped to cope artfully with life's challenges?

You guessed it: they have a level of Mental Fitness that allows them to artfully ride out such things. The greater your Mental Fitness level, the greater your mental and emotional capacity, and the greater your capacity for living happily-despite the curve balls life throws your way.

Clearly, this immunity to being buffeted by life's ups and downs seems to be more naturally developed in some people than others.

And it's true, some people seem to be born with a natural ability to artfully weather life's challenges-that is to say, they are endowed with a higher than average Mental Fitness level. But-and this is crucial-this in no way is to say that one's Mental Fitness level is fixed.

Again, we can take clues from the physical realm. For the same is true of our innate physical fitness levels. Some of us are natural born athletes, others are anything but.

Despite the fact that we humans come in shapes and sizes and physical abilities, no matter what one's natural level of physical fitness is, we ALL can benefit from exercising our physical selves-and improve our physical fitness and live healthier, happier lives.

And so it goes with Mental Fitness.

This means that we are not victims of our natural level of mental fitness, nor of our circumstances. Remember, the greater our Mental Fitness, the easier we can remain undisturbed by the inevitable difficulties that life throws our way. So it paves the way for more happiness and contentment-in good times and bad.

And just as importantly, developing ourselves in this regard can serve as an important component in the health of our communities. Physical fitness aids to stave off physical illness. Mental Fitness aids to stave off mental illness. It's a simple means to enhance the well-being of us all.

With this understanding, the problem becomes one of increasing our Mental Fitness - our capacity to remain mentally and emotionally undisturbed in more and varied circumstances, especially in situations that have historically thrown us off balance.

## *How do I increase my Mental Fitness?*

So, this all begs the question: "How do we increase our Mental Fitness level?" Surprisingly, it's more simple and straightforward than you might think, and truly is not all that different from the way we build more physical fitness.

Think about it. To build our physical capacity, for example your capacity to lift weight, you physically challenge yourself. To lift more weight, you need to lift more weight. Strength builds as you deliberately lift just a bit more weight than you're comfortable with.

If you can easily lift 80 pounds, lift 85; once you can lift 85 without difficulty, move up to 90; and so on. You're expanding your capacity for weight lifting by always lifting just a bit more than is comfortable and by staying with the burn.

The same principle applies when you're working to expand your mental and emotional capacity. Here, too, the plan remains the same: do a bit more than is comfortable and stay with the burn. But for the expansion of our mental and emotional capacity, rather than needing physical weights to provide the resistance needed for growth, we need difficulty or challenge.

Here's the thing: life's challenges, the ones that typically throw us into a tizzy, are for our Mental Fitness, like the weight is to our physical fitness. They are challenges that can be used to increase our capacity to calmly weather life's challenges-but only if we see the opportunities for what they are.

I confess. There is much more nuance to effectively increasing our Mental Fitness levels than is presented in this simplistic explanation. Nevertheless, the premise remains sound. And this I know from experience.

Over the years I've seen dozens of people forge lives of great equanimity and fulfillment even amidst torrents of disappointment and challenges.

My chosen tools are drawn from the ancient wisdom of yoga (tapping the lesser-known mental and emotional aspects of the practice beyond mere yoga postures and breath), but that is not to say these are the only tools that can be used to this end.

Is this orientation toward Mental Fitness a silver bullet?

Will it end mental illness and completely stave off future killings and other such tragedies? Not by a long shot. For the truth is that Mental Fitness can't completely eradicate mental illness any more than physical fitness can totally end physical illness.

We will always have a need for treatment modalities, facilities, and trained professionals to address the needs of those who have slid into mental illness. Just as we do for those who are physically ill.

But if we could take steps to reduce the incidence of such illness even 5 or 10 or 20 percent, wouldn't it be worth it?

The invitation here is to look at the tremendous impact that forging greater physical fitness has had on reducing physical illness. And then orient toward employing those same principles as a means to increasing our Mental Fitness to help reduce the incidence mental illness as well.

## *Depression*

Men must cope with several kinds of stress as they age. If they have been the primary wage earners for their families and have identified heavily with their jobs, they may feel stress upon retirementloss of an important role, loss of self-esteem that can lead to depression. Similarly, the loss of friends and family and the onset of other health problems can trigger depression.

Depression is not a normal part of aging. Depression is an illness that can be effectively treated, thereby decreasing unnecessary suffering, improving the chances for recovery from other illnesses, and prolonging productive life. However, health care professionals may miss depressive symptoms in older patients. Older adults may be reluctant to discuss feelings of sadness or grief, or loss of interest in pleasurable activities.

They may complain primarily of physical symptoms. It may be difficult to discern a co-occurring depressive disorder in patients who present with other illnesses, such as heart disease, stroke, or cancer, which may cause depressive symptoms or may be treated with medications that have side effects that cause depression.

If a depressive illness is diagnosed, treatment with appropriate medication and/or brief psychotherapy can help older adults manage both diseases, thus enhancing survival and quality of life.

Identifying and treating depression in older adults is critical. There is a common misperception that suicide rates are highest among the young, but it is older white males who suffer the highest rate.

Depressive disorders can make one feel exhausted, worthless, helpless, and hopeless. It is important to realize that these negative views are part of the depression and do not accurately reflect the actual circumstances.

Negative thinking fades as treatment begins to take effect. In the meantime: Engage in mild exercise. Go to a movie, a ballgame, or participate in religious, social, or other activities.

Set realistic goals and assume a reasonable amount of responsibility.

Break large tasks into small ones, set some priorities, and do what you can as you can.

Try to be with other people and to confide in someone; it is usually better than being alone and secretive.

Participate in activities that may make you feel better.

Expect your mood to improve gradually, not immediately. Feeling better takes time. Often during treatment of depression, sleep and appetite will begin to improve before depressed mood lifts.

Postpone important decisions. Before deciding to make a significant transition-change jobs, get married or divorced-discuss it with others who know you well and have a more objective view of your situation.

Do not expect to 'snap out of' a depression. But do expect to feel a little better day by day.

Remember, positive thinking will replace the negative thinking as your depression responds to treatment.

Let your family and friends help you.

How Family and Friends Can Help

The most important thing anyone can do for a man who may have depression is to help him get to a doctor for a diagnostic evaluation and treatment. First, try to talk to him about depression help him understand that depression is a common illness among men and is nothing to be ashamed about.

Perhaps share this book with him. Then encourage him to see a doctor to determine the cause of his symptoms and obtain appropriate treatment.

Occasionally, you may need to make an appointment for the depressed person and accompany him to the doctor. Once he is in treatment, you may continue to help by encouraging him to stay with treatment until symptoms begin to lift (several weeks) or to seek different treatment if no improvement occurs.

This may also mean monitoring whether he is taking prescribed medication and/or attending therapy sessions. Encourage him to be honest with the doctor about his use of alcohol and prescription or recreational drugs, and to follow the doctor's orders about the use of these substances while on antidepressant medication.

The second most important thing is to offer emotional support to the depressed person. This involves understanding, patience, affection, and encouragement. Engage him in conversation and listen carefully. Do not disparage the feelings he may express, but point out realities and offer hope.

A man can experience depression in many different ways. He may be grumpy or irritable, or have lost his sense of humor. He might drink too much or abuse drugs. It may be that he physically or verbally abuses his wife and his kids.

He might work all the time, or compulsively seek thrills in high risk behavior. Or, he may seem isolated, withdrawn, and no longer interested in the people or activities he used to enjoy.

Perhaps this man sounds like you. If so, it is important to understand that there is a brain disorder called depression that may be underlying these feelings and behaviors. It's real: scientists have developed sensitive imaging devices that enable us to see depression in the brain.

And it's treatable: more than 80 percent of those suffering from depression respond to existing treatments, and new ones are continually becoming available and helping more people. Talk to a healthcare provider about how you are feeling, and ask for help.

Or perhaps this man sound like someone you care about. Try to talk to him, or to someone who has a chance of getting through to him. Help him to understand that depression is a common illness among men and is nothing to be ashamed about. Encourage him to see a doctor and get an evaluation for depression.

For most men with depression, life doesn't have to be so dark and hopeless. Life is hard enough as it is; and treating depression can free up vital resources to cope with life's challenges effectively.

When a man is depressed, he's not the only one who suffers. His depression also darkens the lives of his family, his friends, virtually everyone close to him. Getting him into treatment can send ripples of healing and hope into all those lives.

Depression is a real illness; it is treatable; and men can have it. It takes courage to ask for help, but help can make all the difference.

*Anxiety*

There's a major difference between the normal, explainable types of anxiety and intense, often crippling anxieties that aren't so easy to explain or understand. Doctors call these "anxiety disorders."

It's estimated that 10 percent of North Americans will experience one of these disorders at some point in their lives. In the past doctors believed that these disorders were directly related to deep-seated psychological problems. Now researchers are finding that genetics and subtle imbalances in brain chemistry may play a significant role.

Anxiety And Depression

The link between anxiety and depression is well known. About 80 percent of people who have been diagnosed with major depression suffer from high levels of anxiety, and about 35 percent of those with anxiety disorders will develop depression.

While most psychiatrists still believe that anxiety and depression are separate illnesses, the diseases often overlap, especially in older adults.

While older people frequently report anxiety as a symptom, they are less likely to suffer from anxiety disorders than people under age 65. Certain negative experiences associated with aging may make you more vulnerable to anxiety.

These include the loss of loved ones, the fear of increased dependency due to health problems, changes in economic or social status, loneliness and fear of isolation, and finally, the fear of dying.

Most people find they can recover from the effects of change and loss if they have enough time. But these stresses tend to pile up in the later years, and it's easy for you to become overwhelmed.

Some experts think that the so-called "young old" people in their 60s and 70s are most vulnerable to anxiety because they are still adjusting to the realities of older age.

Those in their 80s and 90s may actually be less prone to anxiety because longer exposure to loss and stress has given them a measure of resistance.

Common symptoms of Anxiety

* Physical symptoms trembling, twitching or feeling shaky, muscle tension, aches or soreness, pain or discomfort in the chest, shortness of breath, palpitations, sweating, cold or clammy hands, dry mouth, dizziness or lightheadedness, nausea, diarrhea or stomach complaints, flushes or chills, frequent urination, a lump in the throat.

* Emotional symptoms feeling edgy or nervous, easily fatigued, abnormally focused on surroundings or physical sensations, easily startled or upset, trouble concentrating, irritability.

Some Natural Ways To Reduce Anxiety

Yoga is not only an excellent exercise but can reduce it. Having done yoga myself and speaking to some of the group, some of the older men said they joined to relieve anxiety and stress.

These men were there before I joined and they said not only did it work for them, they were so happy that they don't want to stop. As for me, I think I joined just to look at the girls/women. The sa e reason I always joined group activities. □

If yoga is not your cup of tea, try doing your own exercises. It's good for stress and anxiety, because it releases endorphins, nature's way of making you feel better.

Hypnosis is also a very good natural remedy. You can also learn to perform it on yourself after initially seeing a hypnotherapist. There are some really good, affordable products you can use to help you do this on your own. Check out YouTube, you will find lots of video's on how to do self-hypnosis.

Proper abdominal breathing can also be very helpful in reducing it. It takes practice and can be a pain to do, but once you start and get used to it, you'll probably notice the difference.

# CHAPTER 7

## *STUDY, STUDY AND STUDY SOME MORE*

As we age, our mental capabilities decline. However, we do not have to let it happen without a struggle. Seniors that stay mentally active appear to resist the effects of aging of the brain as opposed to their complacent and inactive companions.

Activities that are noted to help increase retention and maintain sharpness include reading books and magazines, doing puzzles such as crosswords, Jumble, and Sudoku, playing games such as Scrabble, using a computer, learning or playing a musical instrument and attending speeches, concerts, lectures and meetings.

Exercise also plays an important role. Those that remain physically active seem to do much better mentally when tested as compared to idle or sedentary seniors.

Watching too much television has a hypnotizing effect and puts the brain into a passive mode which provides much less mental activity than participating in group activities such as discussion groups, taking outdoor walks, riding a bike, aerobic classes, swimming or even dancing.

Seniors that feel appreciated and had the opinion that they had something to contribute tend to maintain their mental capabilities later in life. Many seniors now decide to continue working well into their seventies because they feel that they have the skills and ability to continue to contribute to their jobs or vocations.

Retirement no longer means a decline in activity or occupation. Many people reach their retirement and use it to change their vocation to something that they have always wanted to do but either never had the time or the money to pursue it.

Some decide to do volunteer work and some decide to open their own business. One such individual decided that instead of moving into a retirement community with "a bunch of old folks" he used his retirement savings and opened an antique car restoration business.

Growing old no longer means you are becoming useless. Stay active and you can use your experiences after you retire for something you have always wanted to do.

## Keep your mind busy

We as people for the most part would seldom give this question much thought. It's just not considered the norm for the majority to rate or monitor the sharpness of our mind.

The truth be known most of us allow way too much un-necessary clutter into our mind daily. The media is constantly bombarding us with news of everything that's wrong across the globe. More than likely we are surrounded by negativity daily, even in our own homes.

Chances are if you are an entrepreneur then you are continuously coming across all sorts of information online. As a matter of fact, we all do. The internet is certainly a huge element to keep the mind very busy.

My question to you is, what type of busyness are you allowing your mind to consume. Is it good or bad? Keeping your mind sharp is a very important goal to strive for.

Do you know there are statistics and reports that confirms a record number of people never pick up a book to read after graduating from high school? Other reports show that a mind being idle or not consistently learning new things could be the reason so many people develop Alzheimer's.

Leaders are readers. You hear this saying quite often in the personal development-network marketing arena. That statement holds a lot of truth. Leaders certainly are readers. They feed their mind on growth and personal development materials that's going to sharpen, not only their mind, but skills and relationships, businesses and so forth.

Leaders keep in check the health of their minds by saturating it daily with good quality reading books and audios and by surrounding themselves with likeminded audiences.

If you want to take your mind health to a new level, I suggest you do what all the great leaders are doing and that is daily connecting to the right groups of people and systems. They listen to mentors and coaches, they attend training via webinar or in person. Leaders weed out the negative influences from their lives.

It is very simple to keep our mind sharp. The difficult part is subjecting ourselves to be disciplined enough to execute the task. Simply by becoming aware of your environment, limiting yourself to negativity, keeping your mind busy with good materials that will help you develop in positive ways is the key.

By exercising these good habits, will surely make it much easier to keep a watch over the health of your mind. By doing so the mind becomes more sharper and you will find yourself reaching some of your goals much easier.

## *Ways to Handle Stress and Keep Your Mind Calm*

Stress this era has become the essential component of everyone's life. In fact, it is the most crucial part of every individual's life. You might be wondering why such statement is made. But, wouldn't you agree when I say there is no day in everyone's life when we do not worry?

But as we all know 'worrying' will not help by any means and definitely is not the solution. These are good and easy words to say but hard to believe, when we are stressed we are and we can't really help the mental imbalance.

Here are a few ways that can help you keep calm when you are stressed. These tips are seriously stupid but if you do follow them you will overcome stress scenarios soon.

1. Take a deep long breath.

2. Switch on your air conditioner and your music player and listen to some soothing music. The best would be to listen to rain drops music.

3. Listen to a motivational speaker if you are feeling low and get yourself inspired.

4. Go for a long drive with your family or close friends and ensure you are forgetting your stress as the moment of the long drive passes.

5. Dancing your stress to glory is a great practice too. Many professionals today join dance schools to learn Salsa, Ballroom, Hip Hop etc with intention to not just learn but also keep themselves calm.

6. Count 1 - 20 when you are stressed. Usually inspirational speakers would tip you to count 1 - 10 but I have extended the horizon with the motive to DE-stress completely.

7. Eat Ice Creams or Chocolates when you are stressed as they melt in your mouth your stress melts too. Watch your A1C's!

8. Control your thoughts by reading/listening to some motivational books or books filled with humor content that can add a lot of peace to your stressed mind.

9. Play Puzzles or mind games or even solotaire that can deviate you from the negative thoughts or the stressful thoughts.

10. If you are stressed because of excessive an workload then take a break from work and corner yourself in the workplace for a power nap. Your power nap can last from 15 to 25 minutes but don't sleep it might risk your job. When I as in the Navy we called these "Nooners."

11. At times the stress can be because of the bad behavior of a colleague or someone close to you. The situation is tough to handle, but all you need to do it just take a deep long breath and have a smile on your face and have some motivating thoughts reciting in your mind.

12. Stretching yourself is another way to get a quick relief from the stress. So move away from the stressful scene stretch your body completely for at least 10 minutes you might obtain few

moments of relief. Do cats ever look stressful? A connection to stretching?

13. Surfing Social Media sites could also be a smart practice to deviate your negative thoughts. Accessing Facebook, Twitter and checking the trending topic and following the discussions is fascinating and exciting thing to do.

The above are a few ways that you can handle stress. Control thoughts and keep your mind at peace.

### *Solve puzzles be it crossword or mysteries*

Throughout the ages, puzzles have been important parts of our human experience. A puzzle is merely a problem, a simple question, or a challenge. It is intended to challenge the mind, our senses and our ingenuity to solve complicated problems either in logistical or mathematical nature. Successful resolution can sometimes be attributed to mathematics.

One of the most popular types of puzzles to have ever graced the world is the Jigsaw puzzle. Its origins have been dated to around 1760 where a London-based map maker and engraver decided to mount a map on wood, cut it and used it in teaching geography to children.

The idea became a hit and ever since, jigsaw puzzles have become essential educational tools, even today. Of course, the wealth of puzzles for educational purposes has become expansive and now, there are unique kinds of puzzles to test kids. Some puzzles are open-ended while others offer a specific conclusion.

The Rubik's cube has become one of the most popular puzzles in the 20th century. It was developed in 1974 by Hungarian professor, Erno Rubik. Its popularity and unique challenge to the user has become a sensation especially in the 1980s.

Before, the main goal of solving the Rubik›s cube is to match all same colored tiles on all sides, but then, speed was included in the equation, amplifying the challenge and even today, competitions are being held dedicated to solving the cube in record time.

Word puzzles come in all forms, providing groups of people and individual players a fun activity or past time at home, school or work.

From crossword puzzles, word finding puzzles, and pictograms, from ancient times to the information age, word puzzles are still highly popular especially for English-speaking populations. A lot of regional adaptations have been made throughout the years.

The popularity of puzzles paved way to tons of adventure, suspense and action movies and games. From the death-defying puzzles games in notable games like Tomb Raider, the adventures of Indiana Jones, to the mystery clues of Sherlock Holmes, the idea of problem solving has been reinvented several times, creating an almost cynical look at the world today.

Complexities of puzzles are highly used in Hollywood films and are also adapted in numerous games. There is a challenge in creating a puzzle and when executed flawlessly, gives both the creator and the player an exhilarating experience.

## *Brain Exercises To Improve Memory*

The brain contains everything that makes us who we are. This comprises not only every talent and skill, but also the records of all our experiences, hopes and dreams, the friendships and achievements that give meaning and purpose to our lives.

It's no wonder then, that with every little 'brain hiccup' - forgetting a name, losing our car or house keys (again), a sudden losing streak in our Bridge or Mahjong game - we see our lives slipping away. In fact, many people fear losing their memories more than death itself.

The good news is that although the brain does shrink with age, its remaining capacity is very large. Even with age, most brains can still learn and add new stores of information.

Moreover, there are techniques that show you how to increase brain power and maximize your mental abilities. You can train your brain and improve the efficiency of your memory, whatever your age.

Age and Experience

The common saying 'You can't teach an old dog new tricks' may be catchy but is not true. Ageing may have some effect on memory and learning capacity. However, the experience and knowledge store that age brings can compensate for much of this.

Moreover, memory improvement techniques can help preserve your mental functions into old age. Using simple aids such as diaries, post-it-notes or electronic reminders can also help counter memory slips. I don't know what I would do without my google calendar.

Expand our Interests

As we age, our mental filing cabinets become packed with records of our lives well lived. Yet through it all, the brain makes more complex associations between ideas and puts new learning in the context of a vast store of experience. This means that it becomes easier to take in new information about topics of which we have some knowledge and experience.

So someone who plays chess as a hobby for instance, will build on his knowledge of different chess positions and strategies the more he plays. He can draw on this knowledge and experience when he encounters something similar next time, and become a better player.

The same is true of any area of interest, hobby or profession - Stamp collecting, music, politics, medicine, psychology, astrophysics or even television soap operas. Besides helping to maintain your mental abilities, pursuing a new interest will make life more stimulating.

Two Breakthroughs

The brain, once a mysterious 'black box' that scientists could not decode, is finally revealing some of its biggest secrets. This offers huge promise to anyone who's worried about "losing it". Two of the main findings include

(i) We still grow brain cells

Who doesn't remember downing one too many glasses in their youth and joking, 'Well, there goes another thousand brain cells'? Many of us still believe that we start life with billions of brain cells, and then slowly lose them with time (and alcohol). We'll then have fewer brain cells by our twenties and thirties, and by middle age.

But in fact, in a remarkable discovery, scientists have learned that the brain generates new cells every day, in a process called neurogenesis. What really happens is that most new brain cell growth continues until early adulthood, around the age of 18 to 20.

Thereafter, new brain cells do grow, but more die off than are replaced, so there is a small and gradual but progressive overall loss of brain cells throughout the rest of adulthood.

The crucial point is that it's not the number of cells, but the connections between them that matter. Whenever you learn new things, you create new connections between the cells and thus increase the capacity of your brain.

(ii) The more your use your brain, the greater its capacity

The second major new finding is equally encouraging. We used to think of the brain as if it were a fixed electric power grid, like those that send electricity to our cities.

When the system gets old or overloaded, power decreases which then leads to flickering lights and break down of appliances. We believed that age wore down memory and comprehension in a similar way and there was nothing we could do about it.

Today, we know that the brain can continue to adapt and expand its capacity as needed. Not only does it generate new brain cells bit by bit it also creates new connections between those cells in the form of intricate nerve fibers called dendrites. The more connections in your brain, the faster and better you think.

# CHAPTER 8

*SLEEP. IMPROVE IT.*

Not sleeping enough can weaken the immune system, have a negative effect on your performance of both physical and mental tasks, and even contribute to heart disease. Lack of sleep can impair the memory, too.

As you know, our bodies need a certain amount of sleep in order to function at their best. According to the National Sleep Foundation, an adult who is 65 or older, should get 7 to 8 hours sleep each night while an adult from 26 to 64 years of age may need 7 to 9 hours. Teenagers and school-age children should get even more sleep.

There are four recognized sleep disorders: insomnia, sleep apnea, restless leg syndrome, and narcolepsy. An occasional case of insomnia is normal and could be due to stress, what you ate, jet lag, or other reasons. Insomnia does affect 40% of women and 30% of men.

Sleep apnea is a disorder with interrupted breathing during sleep. Restless leg syndrome could be a disorder common to your family, possibly an inherited trait, and is more common in older people.

Twelve million Americans are affected by restless leg syndrome. Narcolepsy affects about 250,000 Americans. With narcolepsy, people get "sleep attacks" at various times during the day and this is usually hereditary.

As we age, in order to maintain optimum health, the body seems to have a higher requirement for nutrition and exercise. One way to increase nutrition is to add vitamin & mineral supplements.

5% of adults reported having trouble sleeping at one time or another in their life. 64 million Americans regularly suffer from insomnia each year, and 41% more common in women than men.

As we increasingly become more frequent drinkers of caffeine, other factors such as anxiety, excessive use of alcohol or sedatives (sleeping pills for example) changes our sleep pattern's because of shift work or travel also leads to insomnia.

All of us needs to sleep. The record for the longest period without sleep is 18 days, 21 hours, 40 minutes during a rocking chair marathon. The record holder reported hallucinations, paranoia, blurred vision, slurred speech and memory and concentration lapses. It is important that we get get adequate daily sleep as sleeping:

Repairs your body tissues

Helps you recover from your illness

Refreshes your mind

Clears emotional conflicts

Help you perform better at work and at play

The amount of sleep needed varies from one person to another and from one day to the next. As you grow older, you tend to sleep less. That is why our seniors tend to be the earliest to wake up every morning (Not me). When you are sick, you need more sleep. Some women sleep longer during their premenstrual periods.

You don't have to repay your sleep debt hour for hour. You can make up for lost sleep because recovery sleep following sleep deprivation is deeper and of higher quality. Taking sleeping pills produces poorer quality sleep. Also when you take them regularly, you become addicted to them.

In our modern culture, everyday seems to be twice as much work and half as much time to complete it in. Getting a good night's sleep enables us to act and think at our best. Getting a good night's sleep means:

## Breathing Right for Holistic Health and Living

It is a myth that breathing is so natural and spontaneous that it does not require special instructions.

The truth of the matter is that breathing plays such a pivotal role in many aspects of life and living that special instructions are needed to ensure its optimal functioning: aesthetic qualities, such as soft skin and a glowing complexion, or even a beautiful singing voice;

Athletic activities, such as competitive sports; psychological well-being, such as emotional wellness, or freedom from anxiety and stress; spiritual disciplines, such as meditation and spiritual enlightenment; and health and healing, such as holistic health and natural healing. The importance of breathing right cannot be overstated.

But what is supposed to be "natural" may not necessarily be correctly done. When a baby is born, it gasps for its first breath, and then learns to breathe naturally. However, in the process of growth and development, the breathing process may become significantly altered or compromised.

To illustrate, the body shape may change as a result of body weight; the body posture may become misaligned due to lifestyle; the lung capacity may become reduced and restricted because of smoking and other health issues--there are many variables during the course of one's life that may have changed one's breathing process, and thus undermining its functions.

On top of all, aging is the most important factor that adversely affects the breathing process: the respiratory function and lung capacity of an average individual peak in his or her mid 20's, and thereafter decline by as much as 20 percent for every decade of his or her life.

As a result, breathing becomes "unnatural" and compromised breathing may have long-term adverse effects on holistic health and living.

Human health is closely connected to breathing right. According to scientific studies, cancer is anaerobic, which means it cannot survive in high levels of oxygen. Heart diseases and high blood pressure are directly linked to shortness of breath and incomplete breaths.

In addition to optimizing health, the human breath also contributes to holistic living. Controlling breathing holds the key to the art of living well. The explanation is that if you know how to control your breaths, you will also know how to control your mind.

Your life is the sum of your thoughts, which are created by your mind; and how you live your life is determined by your perception and interpretation of those thoughts.

Focusing on your breathing--the inhalation and exhalation of each breath with its own rhythm--is instrumental in training your mind for attention and awareness. Concentration on the present moment leads to mindfulness of self and others, which is an indispensable ingredient in the art of living well.

Breathing provides 99 percent of your oxygen supply, which is the most important energy source in human life. On average, an individual takes more than 20,000 breaths a day. However, it is not the number of breaths that counts, but "how" you take them.

To breathe correctly, first and foremost, you must breathe deeply, using your diaphragm muscles, instead of those of your chest. In addition, your breath, rhythmic and not rough, should be taken in through your nose, and not through your mouth.

To practice diaphragm breathing, sit comfortably in an erect position, placing one hand on your chest and the other on your abdomen.

Begin inhaling through your nose while slightly distending your abdomen; you will feel the movement of your hand over the abdomen, not the one over your chest. Let the air slowly fill up your chest.

Then slowly exhale, without undue exertion, pushing the air out of your lungs down to the abdomen; your hand over the abdomen should feel it collapsing slowly. Repeat the process until it becomes second nature to you.

Breath is life. Controlling your breath and breathing right add a new dimension to every aspect of your health and living. Breathing right is holistic health and living.

### *Self-Hypnosis*

Many people want to be more creative. They want to make things or do things that haven't been done before. One way to help in this goal is to use hypnosis.

Now I know what you are thinking. The same thing most people think when they hear hypnosis. You are seeing a dimly lit lounge with a guy in a cheap tuxedo making grown men bark like a dog whenever they say the word biscuit. This does happen, but there is another side to hypnosis.

First off, what is hypnosis?

Webster's Dictionary defines Hypnosis as: a trancelike state that resembles sleep but is induced by a person whose suggestions are readily accepted by the subject.

What this means is that you are put into a relaxed state. When you are in this state you are more susceptible to suggestion. In this state you can be "retrained" to make changes in your behavior.

Hypnosis has been proven to help with a variety of problems, everything from stress management to weight loss. It has also been used as a means for people to get more creative.

Hypnosis is not a cure all; rather it is a piece of a puzzle to help in the achieving of goals. There are many benefits to hypnosis. It is easy to do, is relatively inexpensive, and there have been no negative side effects associated with it.

By entering the hypnotic state you are both very relaxed and focused. When you are in this state you can learn about yourself. You can find out what is stopping you and break through those roadblocks. To put it simply you can unlock the creativity that exists in you.

Let's talk a little about creativity and what it is. Think back to when you were a child. Think of the way you saw a stick on the ground. The possibilities of that stick were endless. It could be a magic wand, or a sword. As we get older that sort of thinking is stifled by time and circumstance.

If you look around you right now, everything was created. At some point in time nothing around you existed. It was created. In today's society creativity is sometimes stifled. Many times there is a "One size fits all" mentality and we end up in a rut. A lot of the time it is incredibly difficult to get out of that rut. That is where hypnosis can help.

While you are under hypnosis you learn on the subconscious level. While you are in this state a therapist can unlock the part of your brain that controls creativity. By using hypnosis to get to this portion of the brain and unlock it your creative ideas will begin to flow. You will become more playful and start seeing things differently.

By using hypnosis to improve your creativity you can start to see the things in the world around you differently. You can tackle a nagging problem in a different way to get a positive result.

That stick can be a sword again instead of just one more piece of yard clutter that you have to pick up. There will be no end to the possibilities once you have used hypnosis to open yourself up to the creativity that exists inside of you.

## *What Are Binaural Beats?*

Binaural beats were discovered in 1839 by a physicist by the name of Heinrich Wilhelm Dove. Heinrich Wilhelm Dove was born on October 6 1803 in Liegnitz, Prussia. He attended the University of Breslau for 3 years where he studied history, philosophy and natural sciences.

He then pursued further education at the University of Berlin from 1824 to 1826, and in 1838, Dove became an associate professor at the University of Königsberg. One year later, he assumed an associate professor position at the world renowned University of Berlin.

Heinrich Wilhelm Dove's influence on the scientific world was such that there is a crater on the moon, the Dove crater, named after him. He was also presented with the Copley Medal in 1853 because of his many achievements.

During his career, Heinrich Wilhelm Dove wrote over 300 different papers on various subjects ranging from meteorology to experimental physics.

In 1839, Heinrich Wilhelm Dove discovered that when two different sounds of two different, but very close, frequencies were sent to each of his subject's ears, the two frequencies created interference in the subject's brain and merged to produce a whole other frequency, or "beat". And this is how binaural beats were born.

Dove discovered that when two sounds of similar frequencies to those of the brain waves were sent to each ear, the brain would automatically adjust its own brain waves to match those frequencies. This phenomenon is called entrainment and is the main working principle of binaural beats.

But, it wasn't until an American biophysicist by the name of Gerald Oster published a paper on the subject of binaural beats in the 1973 edition of Scientific American magazine called "Auditory Beats in the Brain" that binaural beats were introduced to the mainstream.

Since then, thousands and thousands of different studies were conducted on the wondrous effects of binaural beats. They were even referred to as the first "digital pills" because of their amazing therapeutic properties.

Binaural beats can be used to produce certain states of consciousness. Binaural beats can be used to stimulate creativity or to induce a deep state of meditation.

You can modify the binaural beat's frequency multiple times during a session to give the best experience possible to the listener. Binaural beats can also alter the mood of the subject, making binaural beats a potentially powerful cure against depression.

There are binaural beat recordings that are specifically designed to help you focus better. Some are made to induce a state of happiness and tranquility and some can even be used to cure headaches and high blood pressure. Binaural beats are truly revolutionary therapy tools and there is no telling how far this technology can go.

You can find a large variety of binaural beat CDs or even instant download mp3's on the internet and you will absolutely need good headphones to make the best of them. Binaural beats are totally safe and you won't get addicted to them; so you don't need to worry about undesirable side effects.

- A really good source is YouTube they have hundreds of Binaural beats available that are supposedly designed to address many different issues.

All in all, binaural beats are truly an amazing discovery that will probably change the way we look at traditional therapy forever; and their therapeutic properties will probably never cease to amaze us.

### Why You Should Take Valerian Root For Insomnia?

Insomnia is a common complaint in today's fast paced lifestyle. If left untreated though it could lead to more serious health problems such as high blood pressure and daytime drowsiness. Valerian has been used for hundreds of years as far back as the middle ages to aid sleep.

If you take Valerian root for insomnia you are taking a natural and effective supplement that doesn't have the often unpleasant side effects of sleeping pills. However unlike sleeping tablets Valerian can take a while to show any real effects.

It's best to take Valerian in the evening prior to going to bed. Don't take it if you are driving as it may cause drowsiness. Valerian root can be taken as tea and provides a very soothing and calming drink. The main part of the plant is used to make tablets.

One main benefit of taking valerian is that you aren't putting chemicals into your body which can make you feel a bit hungover the next morning. They could also interfere with other medication or may be dangerous if you are pregnant. Sleeping pills can also become addictive and even make your insomnia worse if you stop taking them.

Valerian increases the levels of GABA in the brain, an amino acid that occurs naturally in the body and lowers the levels of anxiety, giving you a feeling of calm. A lack of GABA can make you feel panicky and stressed. It's also used in medication to help people manage anxiety and can aid sleep

Valerian root is also good for easing joint and muscle pain, and can help to relieve headaches. It's grown in Southern Europe and some areas of North America.

There are many causes of insomnia including anxiety and nervous tension which can be a result of problems at work or with relationships and families. Apart from valerian there are other ways to unwind including a warm milky drink or a cup of chamomile tea. Avoid drinking coffee in the evening unless it's decaffeinated.

Low levels of melatonin a hormone that promotes sleep and released into the body as dusk falls, can also cause insomnia. As well as valerian you could try taking melatonin as it's also available as a supplement. This applies if you are working shifts or frequently take long haul flights.

So take valerian root for insomnia and after a few weeks or less you will begin to notice you are sleeping better and also feel calmer.

# CHAPTER 9

## *SUPPLEMENT OR NOT TO SUPPLEMENT.*

Sometimes we are guilty of having more than what is necessary and that is because we often get carried away by two things: hype and the desire to keep up with everyone else. We fail to realize that it is in our best interest to get only what we need and not what we want because the latter tends to get us in more trouble than we can handle.

The same can be said when deciding whether to take supplements or not. Bodybuilders in particular, are the ones who are said to need supplements best because of the intense training and workout routines they do to build muscles and get that ripped physique.

They also require supplements because the diet they put themselves on often makes them miss out on other nutritional needs that they can't incorporate into their diet like carbohydrates and fats.

However, there are those who believe that they don't require supplements because they do just fine without it. Their muscles will still grow, their bodies will still shape up and that ripped physique is going to happen with perseverance and dedication, which means no slacking off. So why do people still tend to think that supplements are important and that they should be taken?

Again, this is where hype comes in. Once a product gets rave reviews from experts, namely famous bodybuilders or celebrities with toned and buff bodies, people are ready to scramble and get themselves the same supplements apparently used by this and that famous person and expect the same results to happen to them.

Alas, most of the time, we end up being disappointed and more than just a bit disillusioned that a miracle hasn't happened.

The first thing you need to realize is that supplements aren't mandatory. In bodybuilding, anyone who works and trains hard, and consumes the right amounts of protein, carbohydrates and fats will achieve their fitness goals in time. But, if their goal is to become big and strong as they possibly can, then yes, they should take supplements to help them maximize their workouts for optimum results.

Going through training and workouts as intense as those of bodybuilders' can make your body weak, plus, you can experience nutritional deficiencies because your energy is used up quickly. Bodybuilders need to take supplements to help them stay healthy during their workouts and to help their body burn fat efficiently.

Also, if you want to maximize your muscle gain and achieve a certain size and level of strength, then supplements are something that you should take, particularly those with whey protein, creatine, glutamine, high-potency multivitamins and essential fatty acids.

So to answer the question of whether or not bodybuilders should take supplements or not, the answer is no, they don't need to but if they want to get maximum results out of their hard work at the gym, then yes, they should take supplements.

As long as you follow the required dosages and follow both your doctor and product recommendations, you should be fine. Also, remember that supplements aren't truly worth your time and money unless they work for you, so when you do buy supplements, make sure you do research and buy what you really need.

# CHAPTER 10

*HORMONE HEALTH*

We all know that exercise is important; there are many benefits of exercise like - cardiovascular health and overall stress management. But exercise is more than maintaining cardiovascular health.

Studies on exercise have indicated that engaging in moderate exercise, meaning a brisk walk, 3x a week for 20 minute intervals, is beneficial for supporting hormonal balance, immune system function, cognitive ability and breathing disorders in addition to the many benefits seen for cardiovascular health.

In fact, if one looked at the studies surrounding exercise, it becomes apparent that exercise may be the best preventative strategy for living a long and healthy life. Let's take a look at what a moderate exercise program can do for the human body.

Hormonal Health

Moderate 30 minute exercise programs have been shown to improve stress levels and increase coping ability and these benefits seem to extend to tai chi and yoga based exercise programs and not only cardiovascular or strength based programs

We also know a lot more about the hormonal effects of activity and exercise now and a 21st Century exercise program is all about restoring body composition (muscle/fat ratio) to a healthy balance.

This cannot be achieved by any type of 'cardio' type activity. Our muscle tissue makes up to 50 percent of our body weight and its health and condition determines the level of our health right through adulthood.

If you allow your muscles to become weak, flabby and wither away from lack of use you are taking a big risk with your health and ultimately your life. It is so easy to fit in 2-3 sessions of strength training each week. Even this small amount is a powerful efficient tool that will work at keeping your hormone levels in a better balance.

This will give you more youthful strength, vitality, vigor and energy than you may have had in years (maybe decades. So, get yourself started as the sooner you do the sooner you can enjoy the many benefits this old but proven form of exercise can give you.

Immune System Function

Exercise is highly beneficial for immune system health and moderate exercise has been shown to stimulate immune cell production, elevate temperatures to assist in the removal of bacterial agents, increase excretion of carcinogens and encourage early detection of viral infections.

Exercise also modulates the stress response and controls inflammation in immune based episodes and appears to decrease both the duration as well as the severity of influenza (Flu) infections.

Exercise also appears to decrease the prevalence of infections for those participating in moderate exercise and increases antibody response in response to vaccinations.

Memory and Cognitive Function

While there is a lack of research in this area, studies do indicate that moderate exercise programs reduce the risk of dementia for some individuals and that individuals with the lowest levels of exercise participation may be twice as likely to develop dementia conditions compared to those with higher levels of exercise participation.

Research also indicates that exercise, in conjunction with a healthy diet, moderate alcohol intake and smoking cessation, may provide the greatest protection against the development of dementia.

Science is constantly updating our knowledge about our health and wellness. One of the areas that we know more about and has become big business in the last decade or so is our hormonal health. Our hormones are the chemical messengers that give instructions to our cells and systems.

We know now that when we get sick particularly if we get a chronic disease that it is related to unfavorable changes in our hormonal levels. Millions of people are hospitalized and many die each year because of the shifts in these levels that trigger other changes that lead to dozens of diseases that make us sick.

The degenerative process that we know as aging gives us the wrinkles, the stooped posture and the grey hair. What it also gives us that is not so visible is dwindling muscle tissue and bone strength, an increase in excess body fat, a decrease in the efficiency of our body systems and processes, lowered energy levels and a susceptibility to disease.

This is the dreaded downward spiral of aging which if we let it sucks us into its clutches. It can take us from a strong, energetic and vital being into a state of weakness and feebleness which leads to the sad disability we see in old people in the last third of their life. Along with this decline come apathy and little desire to be active which further hastens the 'shutdown mode'.

But it does not have to be this way; we know now through research that our hormonal levels can be improved with the stimulation that comes from being physically active. But not just pottering around the house active - that will not even come close to cutting it.

What is needed is a strength training exercise program that is designed to rebuild and tone up muscle tissue that in turn will stimulate 'growth and repair' hormones that will improve health, slow down the aging process and boost the immune system to protect us from disease.

## The Dangers of Hormonal Imbalance

Hormonal disorder is associated with distressing and irritating symptoms such depression, insomnia, panic attacks, memory loss, weight gain, pain, and several other forms of discomfort.

Although hormonal change can be brought about by age, an abusive lifestyle is what worsens the whole thing. People who keep themselves fit and healthy tend to age more gracefully.

They are not so anxious about aging. Specifically, the amount of alcohol and the type of food that you eat affects your hormones. Besides, health problems like fatigue, Thyroid, or insulin imbalance may also influence the functionality of your hormones.

The ill effects of hormonal imbalance are not only experienced by women, but by men too. As men grow older, their testosterone levels fall while their estrogen levels rise.

Sometimes, older men may have higher estrogen levels compared to their female counter parts of the same age. Furthermore, men may also suffer from urinary problems, erectile dysfunction, and low sperm count.

In fact, if immediate action is not taken, they may have to deal with bigger problems such as cancer. Why would you want to wait until things turn that nasty? You have many things you can do now to avoid going through that kind of experience in your near future.

So what are some of the options available for us now to escape the misery associated with hormonal imbalance? First is to learn how to make wise decisions.

Some wisest decisions you can make include: leading a healthier lifestyle, having enough rest and doing exercise regularly. As far as diet is concerned, ensure that enough vegetables, vitamins and minerals are on your daily menu.

You will certainly feel and look great if your body maintains a proper hormonal balance. To maintain that balance, you need to continuously ensure that you avoid taking in lots of toxins in your body. At the end of the day, you will realize that your mind is always active and alert to handle the most difficult moments you go through in your daily routine.

Remember you don't have to wait until it's too late to act. Some people only wake up on realizing that their hormonal count has hit its lowest. That can be very harmful to your health. You need to act immediately to restore your health so that you can still do the things you enjoy doing.

Resorting to hormonal replacement with artificial substitutes is not the most effective solution as it tends to have many side effects harmful to your health.

Going the natural way is the most safe and effective solution to fixing a hormonal imbalance crisis. Therapy from an expert can be an option as long as you are confident there wont be any damages to your overall system.

## Hormone Replacement Therapy

An imbalance of hormones can cause a range of psychological and physiological symptoms. People generally produce fewer hormones as they age, and hormonal deficiencies may also result from environmental and nutritional factors.

Restoring hormones to their proper balance often improves a person's health and overall happiness.

Physicians achieve this goal with hormone replacement therapy (HRT), which supplements a person's natural supply of hormones such as estrogen and testosterone. Men and women may both receive HRT, although the specific benefits and effectiveness differ between the sexes.

HRT may refer to any type of therapy in which the patient receives hormones as medical treatment. This includes supplements of naturally-occurring hormones as well as the substitution of similar hormones. HRT generally has three forms, including HRT for menopause, androgen replacement therapy and HRT for transgender people.

The purpose of HRT for menopause is to reduce the symptoms caused by a reduction in the levels of estrogen and progesterone in the bloodstream. This commonly occurs during menopause, although women who have their ovaries removed also have a lower estrogen level.

Androgen replacement therapy (ART) sometimes called Testosterone Replacement Therapy (TRT) is primarily used to supplement a man's natural testosterone. This is generally the result of hypogonadism, in which a man's testes don't produce sufficient amounts of testosterone. Various conditions such as cancer can cause hypogonadism, and it's also a natural part of the aging process.

Bio-identical hormone replacement therapy (BHRT) is a type of HRT that uses hormones that are molecularly identical to the ones used in traditional HRT. The goal of this form of HRT is generally to achieve a desired hormone level, as measured by blood or saliva testing.

Hormones commonly used in BHRT include estradiol, estrone and progesterone, which are commonly available in manufactured products and products compounded at a pharmacy.

BHRT may use dehydroepiandrosterone and testosterone, although the availability of these products is more limited in North America. Estriol is also available in Europe for BHRT.

Administration

Physicians may administer HRT with a variety of methods including injections, pellets, pills, patches and creams. They will routinely adjust the specific dosage and approach to provide maximum benefits with minimal side effects. It›s therefore essential for patients to report any side effects when receiving HRT.

Pellets

Pellets are inserted under the skin, where they release a consistent dose of hormones over a period of time, typically at least four months. This administration method is most often used in BHRT with pellets that contain hormones from natural sources such as plants.

Pellets create smaller fluctuations in hormone levels compared to other administration methods, which can result in a roller coaster effect as the hormone level rises and falls.

Patches and Creams

Therapists also use patches to deliver a variety of hormones, including estrogen and testosterone. The patch then delivers the hormone into the bloodstream at a specific rate. The patch is typically applied by the patient to the buttocks or abdomen for up to one week. The patient may then remove the old patch and apply a new one. A patch remains on at all times, even while bathing or swimming.

Testosterone

Testosterone is a hormone that belongs to the androgen group and is also the primary male sex hormone. The testes of male mammals produce testosterone, as does the ovaries of females. The adrenal glands also produce testosterone, although in smaller amounts.

Testosterone causes the masculizing effects that occur in boys during puberty, and some of these changes begin to reverse themselves when a man's testosterone production declines during middle age.

This condition is sometimes known as andropause, although this term is not currently recognized as a medical classification by the World Health Organization.

ART may use testosterone as well as synthetic androgens such as nandrolone. It can be self-administered by the patient using various means such as creams, gels, pills, tablets and patches. A physician may also administer ART by injecting the androgen deep into the patient's fat or muscle. I currently use the injection method and do this myself at home once a week.

Benefits for Men

A man's testosterone production normally declines as he enters middle age, which often produces the following categories of symptoms:

Physical changes

Emotional changes

Sexual dysfunction

The physical changes caused by a reduced testosterone level typically include a loss of muscle mass and strength. It can increase the amount of body fat, especially abdominal fat. It may also decrease bone density and cause the skin to become thinner. Hair loss, fatigue and hot flashes are symptoms that may occur in middle-aged men.

Additional symptoms of a low testosterone level include tender, swollen breasts, known medically as gynecomastia. Low testosterone may also cause sleeping difficulties such as insomnia, and it's a risk factor for type II diabetes and metabolic syndrome.

Emotional changes associated with low testosterone in men include a loss of self-confidence and motivation. It can also create feelings of depression and sadness. A low testosterone level can cause some men to experience difficulty with memory and concentration.

Sexual problems are also a common result of low testosterone. The may include a reduction in the frequency of spontaneous erections and a loss of sexual desire. Erectile dysfunction and infertility are more severe sexual problems caused by lower testosterone.

The development of ART is primarily the result of dissatisfaction with the male aging process. Hypogonadism is common in older men, although it's frequently undiagnosed and rarely treated. A 2008 study in PostGraduate Medicine reports strongly consistent evidence that ART is effective in restoring a man's loss of sexual function and body composition due to low testosterone.

The evidence for ART's effectiveness in restoring bone density is moderately consistent. The evidence for reducing the patient's sensitivity to insulin, lipid levels and glycemic control is inconsistent. The evidence that ART can improve a patient's cognitive function and mood is weakly inconsistent.

*Naturally Declining Testosterone Levels*

A few men have less than normal androgenic hormone or testosterone levels without indications of it. For others, reduced testosterone may cause dramatic alterations in sexual function including reduced sexual interest, fewer spontaneous occurrences of erections - such as while asleep - and the inability to conceive.

Further, sleep sometimes can be affected with the reduced testosterone causing sleeplessness or other disturbances to rest.

In fact, the entire body can be changed such as increased body fat, decreased muscle bulk as well as a loss of strength and endurance together with reduced bone density.

Many men also suffer inflamed or tender breasts and pattern baldness and hair thinning is widely known to be related to testosterone levels. Men might experience bursts of body heat or flashes and generally have less than the energy to what they are used to.

But it doesn't stop there. Low androgenic hormone or testosterone may contribute to the decrease in inspiration, motivation and self-confidence. Many men report that they may really feel sad or stressed out, or have difficulty concentrating or recalling things.

It's important to observe that some of these signs or symptoms are a regular part of getting older. Others call this a morbidity trance - where people resign themselves to aging and accept it as a somehow normal. But is it right to be so self-defeated and to allow these conditions related to the body's deterioration?

Others can be brought on by various underlying elements, including medication's unwanted side-effects, thyroid problems, depressive disorders and excessive alcoholic beverages use. A bloodstream test is the only method to diagnose a low androgenic hormone or testosterone level.

When diagnosed, the important thing to remember is that it all can be treated. Doctors will argue for a Hormone replacement therapy, mostly because they get commissions from drug companies. The very real alternative is to consider testosterone boosting dietary supplements.

## How To Raise Testosterone Level With Exercise And Foods

Testosterone, sometimes referred to as the "male hormone" plays a very important role in the development of male reproductive organs such as the testicles and prostates and also in the male characteristics such as increased muscle mass, bone mass, and the growth of bodily hair. This wonder hormone also maintains sex drive and helps to prevent osteoporosis.

Unfortunately, the natural production of testosterone starts to decline as a man gets older with age and most men start to notice a natural decline in their testosterone level during their 40s when they notice that they are gaining belly fat, losing muscle mass, declining sex drive and for some, unable to get erections.

The good news is that apart from the medical procedure of testosterone replacement therapy, there are ways to slow down the declining production or even to raise your testosterone level naturally.

A good combination of the right foods to eat and exercise can promote natural increases in testosterone levels and you can regain your strong and virile self once again.

So how can we increase our testosterone level naturally? Well, get a gym membership and start lifting weights. Train with exercises that incorporate a wide range of body parts such as bench presses, squats and deadlifts to fatigue your body.

That is because due to the fatigue and the metabolic demands those exercises place on your body, your system is forced to produce more testosterone to repair your muscles and strengthen your bones.

For the exercises to be more effective in raising your testosterone level, you must train with intensity. So train hard. Research has shown that when you exercise with maximal exertion and exercising until fatigued, more testosterone is being produced.

When you workout with weights and with compound exercises, you will also fuel muscle growth much faster and this in turn will raise your metabolism and will help you to reduce your belly fat making you less susceptible to heart diseases, stroke, hypertension and diabetes. Training with such intensity is also known to reduce your bad cholesterol and raise your good cholesterol.

The foods that you eat can also help you to raise your testosterone level because these foods contain specific nutrients that help in the production of testosterone.

Fish fat - The fats found in fish, especially cold water fish can increase your testosterone level. Omega 3 fatty acids found in fish fat can increase our HDL level (good cholesterol) which our body uses to produce more testosterone.

Oysters - Good news for oyster lovers. This humble shellfish have been used for centuries by many cultures as an aphrodisiac. This is because oysters contain zinc, which is a potent mineral needed for the production of testosterone.

Red meat - Although red meat can help you to increase your testosterone level, to be more effective, just make sure you are getting grass-fed and hormone injection free red meat.

This is because animals fed the natural way are leaner and are with higher Omega-3 fatty acids. Since they are leaner, then you need not worry about consuming too much saturated fat and eating more calories than is required.

Avocados - Avocados contain vitamin B6 which is helpful in increasing testosterone production. Avocados also have high levels of potassium that assists in regulating the thyroid gland that may help in increasing the male sex drive.

Beans - Beans contain more zinc than any other member of the vegetable family so much so that some beans even rival the zinc content of red meat. Bet you didn›t know that, didn›t you?

Beans are also high in protein and fiber but low in fat, so it is an excellent food to help repair your muscle tissues after your workouts and at the same time keeping you lean and mean.

Supplements - There are also natural supplements available which contain active ingredients that are said encourage your body to produce more testosterone. They are commonly known as testosterone enhancers or boosters. If unsure, just ask your local drugstore pharmacist. Tip: Research DHEA.

So, by eating the right foods and exercising in the right way, you can stay and look younger much longer with an increase surge of testosterone in your body. So start to raise your virile male hormones now and become stronger and sexier.

## *How to Lower Estrogen Levels For Men*

Testosterone is the primary hormone that gives men their "male" characteristics. Once a boy hits puberty his body gets flooded with testosterone and he becomes a man. Testosterone is responsible for the proper development of male sexual characteristics.

It is also important for maintaining muscle bulk, adequate levels of red blood cells, bone density, sense of well-being, and sexual and reproductive function.

On the flip side, women have estrogen, which is the female "equivalent" of testosterone. In women, estrogen is what is responsible for the proper development of female sexual characteristics.

So men have testosterone and women have estrogen, right? Wrong. Men have testosterone and estrogen-women have both too. The difference is that men produce about ten times more testosterone than women do (and vice versa). So though our bodies are dominant in testosterone, we also produce low levels of estrogen.

In fact, a certain amount of estrogen in men is necessary for proper body function. Too little estrogen and we run the risk of developing osteoporosis and other conditions. Too much though and we start developing female characteristics, which is not a good a thing-for health or the ego.

As men age their testosterone levels will naturally start to drop (by about one percent per year). Similarly, their estrogen levels will start to increase.

When estrogen levels start getting high in men, health problems start to arise. Elevated estrogen levels in men have been shown to contribute to prostate cancer and heart disease, along with gynecomastia-also known as "man boobs."

Since higher levels of estrogen are typically accompanied by lower levels of testosterone, other changes occur including loss of muscle mass, fatigue, low libido, erectile dysfunction. Lastly, excessive estrogen in men raises body fat and can contribute to diabetes and high lipids.

But it's not just older guys who experience higher levels of estrogen-it happens to young guys too. Guys who don't take care of themselves are far more likely to show elevated estrogen levels than men who are in good shape. For example, testosterone begins to convert to estrogen in men as they age due to the aromatase reaction.

Aromatase is an enzyme that plays a role in converting testosterone to estrogen and is found most prevalently in fat cells. Therefore, the more body fat a man has the more aromatase and the more estrogen he is likely to have.

So you see, a younger guy who is overweight with excess fat-especially around the middle-will likely see a spike in estrogen levels accompanied by a drop in testosterone levels.

Rule number one to avoid excessive estrogen levels: maintain a healthy body weight-build and maintain lean muscle mass. In particular, pay close attention to the fat around the middle of your body. These fat cells are known to produce aromatase, which can lead to higher estrogen levels in men, thus changing the hormonal balance.

There are plenty of other things that can lead to higher estrogen levels in men too so guys of any age should be aware of the following:

• Medications: Some medications can cause estrogen levels to rise so be on the lookout for estrogen-containing drugs, steroids, ulcer medications such as cimetidine, some antibiotics (tetracycline, ampicillin, etc.), anti-fungal medications and antidepressants. Since there are more medications that can cause this effect, you should check with your doctor or pharmacist.

• Illness: Certain illnesses also cause spikes in estrogen levels including some tumors of the testes, adrenal and pituitary glands, liver and lung, cirrhosis (liver disease). Kidney and thyroid disease may elevate estrogen levels as well.

• Drugs: Using illicit drugs is another sure-fire way to cause a jump in estrogen so stay away from anabolic steroids, marijuana, cocaine and other drugs that can affect hormone levels.

• Alcohol: Moderate drinking generally doesn't cause problems but frequent benders can. Drinking excessively can increase the body's conversion of testosterone into estrogen, especially in fat cells. It can also block the liver from effectively eliminating excess estrogen.

• Environmental exposure: Things that we run across in our daily lives can also contribute to elevated estrogen levels in men. The list of pesticides, chemicals and herbicides that have the potential to cause estrogen-like effects in the body is lengthy so do yourself a favor and avoid them as much as possible.

A number of experts have also begun to believe that there is a link between the ingestion of hormone-enhanced food and elevated estrogen levels. More research is sure to be done on the subject so stay tuned. In any case, hormone- and pesticide-free, unprocessed foods are best for your body so stick with those.

### *How To Build Body Mass and Get A Shredded Physique?*

Building muscle mass means that an individual must do two things and the first is that you must adjust your diet so that you are eating right in order to support and increase in body mass.

Your diet must include foods that are high in protein, high in fiber, and you should increase your carbohydrate levels so that your body has the energy that it needs to build the extra muscle mass. In addition to increasing high protein and high fiber foods, you should begin eliminating foods that are high in fat.

If you are adjusting your diet to help increase body mass you should also be aware that your body will need extra calories. In order to include those needed foods in your diet you will have to carefully plan out your daily meals. If you find it difficult to get just the right blend of healthy mass building foods, you may want to consult a dietician for more advice.

The second thing that you must do in order to increase body mass is that you will need to develop a work out plan that is designed to increase body mass and this means lots of weight lifting.

When building body mass the goal is to increase muscle and not fat and the only way to do this is to physically exercise. Lifting weights as part of your workout routine ensure that the energy your body does have to expend is turned into muscle during exercise.

Building body mass can easily be done if you follow the aforementioned steps and the benefits of increasing the mass are bountiful.

The first benefit of building more mass is of course the fact that you will look so much better physically, but there are many others including increased stamina, easier loss of body fat, and increasing your metabolism. These items combined mean overall you will have a healthier and therefore happier you.

There is equipment designed to build body mass and develop your muscles like weight lifting equipment and equipment, designed to burn fat and loose weight like fitness equipment. Muscular and strength equipment increases the muscles' strength, reduces the level of cholesterol and helps keeping down the levels of blood pressure and sugar.

It is useful to people of any age and condition and may help you to shape your body the way you want.

The muscular and strength exercise equipment includes free weights, dumbbells, barbells, ab training equipment, weight training benches, weight racks, vertical knee raise and dip stations, steps, cable machines, leg equipment such as leg presses, leg curl machines, leg extension machines, calf raises etc.

Free weights come in different sizes and colors and are very easy to use. By using them you increase your muscle endurance, strength, power as well as your bones density and your flexibility. They are portable, not expensive and can be used even in front of the TV.

A type of free weight is the dumbbell. It also varies in size and shape and helps improving the muscle mass on your triceps, shoulders and your chest.

There are Selectric dumbbells (their weight can be changed mechanically not manually, fixed weight dumbbells (dumbbell - shaped weights), adjustable dumbbells (the plates are to be added or removed manually).

Barbells include a set of collars (the metal components that secure the weights in place), a set of weight plates (discs) and a metal bar (usually steel). The bars come in different length and diameter (women's bar is shorter and lighter).

There are standard barbells, Olympic barbells, Triceps bars, EZ Curl Bars, Thick handled Barbells etc. Bear in mind that when lifting barbells you are going to need spotters, for your own safety.

Leg presses are used to strengthen the lower part of the body, especially quadriceps, Gluteus Maximus, calves and hamstrings. Leg presses are leg equipment used to push away a weight by legs.

Leg Extension Machines are used for strengthening the quadriceps muscle. In order to execute the calf raises, you should need a seated or a standing calf raise.

A type of resistance training is the usage of weighted clothing. The lower body weighted clothing includes ankle weights, thigh weights, and weighted footwear.

The Core weighted clothing includes weighted belts, dip belts, hip drags, weight vests, neck weights, head weights, weighted backpacks, and integrated weight systems. The upper body weighted clothing includes upper arm weights, wrist weights, and weighted gloves.

Weight training benches are also weight lifting equipment. They can be fixed inclined, fixed horizontal, with one, two or more adjustable portions, fixed in a folded position etc.

# CHAPTER 11

## *START YOUR FITNESS PROGRAM NOW AND DON'T EVER STOP*

How do you see yourself at age 65? If you are like the average person you will have probably retired from your job - and your exercise routine. Imagine it, a spare tire has settled around your midsection and your knees hurt when you move around.

Your length of stride has reduced to a shuffle and your balance is so poor you have to be careful navigating over something higher than a half an inch. And forget about touching your toes - on a good day you might just reach your shins.

All in all the life force has been sucked out of you like some dwindling old engine. Yes, you will clock up some years as the decades tick by, but you don›t have to watch your health and vitality quietly fade away.

No matter what your current age or physical condition with the right exercise program containing strength training you can regain and maintain an exceptional level of strength and fitness. In fact 6 months of the right exercise can reverse 30 years of inactivity. How's that for reclaiming your youth?

It is important to understand that getting older doesn't mean losing your strength, energy and vitality. Like a good bottle of red wine you can get better with age and you can be stronger and look better at 60 than you did at 30.

Is that likely? Unfortunately if you are like most 50- plus people, you may believe that you are too old to begin a proper exercise program. However if you commit right now to get in about four hours of proper exercise each week - not much, considering the average person watches 20 hours of television weekly - you will see results almost immediately.

Staying strong and breaking into a sweat regularly is a crucial part of becoming and staying a healthy person. Rather than relying on doctors and drugs think of your exercise program as medicine. And this medicine is the most powerful tool you can prescribe for yourself to prevent the many nasty diseases and conditions that may well shorten your life or leave you disabled and unable to care for yourself.

The average person due to their lack of strength and fitness needs around 10 years of care towards the end of their lives just to manage daily tasks of living. With the right exercise this can be reduced down to around 3 years. Wouldn't that be a great gift to give to family, your community and the world?

Why should someone else be responsible for taking up the slack for our care when it could have easily been prevented by each of us taking personal responsibility for our own health and well-being? It is important to believe that what we do right through our lifespan with our strength and fitness determines what happens in the last 15- 20 years of our lives.

Your fifth or sixth decade of life isn't a bad time to start an exercise program. In fact, for many people, the freedom they experience later in life - from having their kids out of the house delivers a powerful impetus and opportunity to make fitness a priority.

This exercise program must be right, don›t think that just going for walk or doing the gardening is going to cut it as it won›t. The program must contain strength building exercise and some low level cardio interval training.

It is crucial that this program is set up, taught, supervised and monitored by a fitness professional. This will ensure that it is safe, progressive and effective.

Whether you are climbing a mountain at 75 or sitting in some rest home somewhere not knowing what your name is and not being able to feed and dress yourself is totally up to what you do right now. The secret: Start wherever you are now, and don't ever stop.

Health, nutrition, fitness and exercise are starting to add themselves to your list of concerns now that you're in your 40's and 50's. It may start with a bit of back pain when you get up in the morning or the first time you find yourself running short of breath after climbing stairs.

And by now you're probably starting to ponder how you'll feel, how much energy you'll have and what you simply won't be able to do in another 20 or 30 years...

Senior health will become more and more important to you as time goes on, and the best time to start making adjustments to help ensure a fit, healthy and enjoyable retirement is right now.

Waiting to address senior health & wellness issues until you're in your 60's and 70's won't be a great idea for you - it would be much like starting your retirement savings plan shortly after retirement. By now you're probably starting to save or invest for that, right? So why do less for your own health & fitness levels when that will play just as big a role in what you can enjoy then?

There is good news and bad news for you now that you're in your 40's or 50's. You're most likely already aware of the bad news - your body's production of important hormones like testosterone and growth hormone are declining, and, left unabated, will keep dropping as you age.

If you're like most people you've been sitting for 8 hours a day or more for decades now, your physical activity levels have been eroded by family, work, societal and financial concerns and you've fallen into the habit of collapsing in front of the TV or computer each night where you'll vegetate for a couple of hours before heading to bed. And even then your 8 hours of restful, uninterrupted sleep is but a fond memory...

The good news is that, in most cases, your body is very willing to forgive your transgressions - but it needs your help, and it needs it starting now before more conditions become irreversible.

# CONCLUSION

The majority of us don't really comprehend our individual health and physical fitness. The fundamentals are sometimes even unidentified. It is always significant to be in shape, all of us has learned this.

Your physical fitness has a huge impact with regards to how you are feeling regarding your physical along with psychological state of mind, and the amount of force your body has to apply in an effort to go on working.

Insufficient physical fitness has supposedly made it to a terrible proportion inside North America, though the fact is that Individuals still are compulsive about health and physical fitness, furthermore primetime physicians plus celebrities alike create an abundance of money due to promoting fitness video tutorials and books for the community.

Unless you are aiming to purchase them altogether and use them as weights to pick up then down day by day, none of these will ever do your bodily fitness any good at all.

The best way to improve your health and physical fitness is by means of incorporating habitual activity into your day by day program. It just isn't necessary to take out full membership at any local fitness center, or merely attend one fitness workout lesson.

Although, what this means is selecting an exercise which increases your heart speed, or improves your strength as well as general mobility.

Doing a quick run, strolling a number of blocks, performing some gardening or chores around the house, walking up and down the steps, are all examples of something whose function is to blend pretty straightforwardly into your routine, however which often also increase your physical health.

On the contrary, jumping on the elevator, driving the auto enroute to the store along at the bend of your boulevard, and spending longer in bed are altogether things that will not improve your fitness level. Make an effort every day to take a stride on the road to improving your own health and physical fitness.

A healthful way of life can't be a fad, otherwise something that you're going to do sometime down the road. It needs to be on your 'to-do' list all year around, not as a New Year Resolution that you simply on no account shall maintain.

After you begin on some sort of workout regime, you will have to maintain this up for the remaining of your days; or else your physical condition is going to be gone, plus you could have to begin all over another time.

With no standard workout, the muscle tissues lessen, afterward extra fat takes its spot (muscle masses will not become fats, they merely push over to make additional space intended for it if they are not in use).

This is consequently essential that you choose a routine with the intention of keeping you interested in the long term; each month bestows the most current 'fitness fad', although almost everyone takes them up and then discards them after a short time. As an alternative, select something that you simply get pleasure from.

And see if the thought of being taught on hopping up then down over a plastic panel fills you with scorn, then you might try something else - martial arts will always be trendy, and then a personal fitness regime which incorporates selected types of team sport will assist to hold your interests.

Keep in mind: personal activity day-to-day is the important thing for fitness, moreover that is what is significant.

Improving your personal form can offer you added energy, as well as will help you feel even more certain about your body.

www.ingramcontent.com/pod-product-compliance
Lightning Source LLC
Chambersburg PA
CBHW031238250726

48655CB00005B/2009